PRAISE FOR FINDING THE SOURCE

"Patients, physicians, nurses, and dentists can all learn something from Dr. Romano. His mind works at an incredible speed and thankfully, he put his thoughts down on paper so you can go at your own pace. *Finding the Source* is an amazing depiction of how an orthopaedic surgeon evaluates his patients to determine the origin of their problem."

— DANIEL G. KLAUER, DDS

"*Finding the Source* is a book with a soul. Dr. Romano's personal search for the causes of injuries can once again take medicine out of the laboratory and place clinical practice as a prime mover in the advancement of healthcare excellence. The patient's concerns and worries have to become the doctor's. I know that is how Dr. Romano approached every patient … after twenty years of working with him, he never once rushed or refused to see a patient. My advice is to read this book."

— JOSEPH C. SHEEHAN, MD

FINDING THE
SOURCE

FINDING THE
SOURCE

Maximizing Your Results—
With and Without
Orthopaedic Surgery

VICTOR M. ROMANO, MD
Board Certified Orthopaedic Surgeon

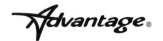

Published by Advantage, Charleston, South Carolina.
Member of Advantage Media Group.

ADVANTAGE is a registered trademark, and the Advantage colophon is a trademark of Advantage Media Group, Inc.

Printed in the United States of America.

10 9 8 7 6 5 4 3 2 1

ISBN: 978-1-59932-910-9
LCCN: 2018933605

Cover and layout design by Carly Blake.

This publication is designed to provide accurate and authoritative information in regard to the subject matter covered. It is sold with the understanding that the publisher is not engaged in rendering medical, legal, accounting, or other professional services. If medical advice or other expert assistance is required, the services of a competent professional person should be sought.

Advantage Media Group is proud to be a part of the Tree Neutral® program. Tree Neutral offsets the number of trees consumed in the production and printing of this book by taking proactive steps such as planting trees in direct proportion to the number of trees used to print books. To learn more about Tree Neutral, please visit **www.treeneutral.com**.

Advantage Media Group is a publisher of business, self-improvement, and professional development books and online learning. We help entrepreneurs, business leaders, and professionals share their Stories, Passion, and Knowledge to help others Learn & Grow. Do you have a manuscript or book idea that you would like us to consider for publishing? Please visit **advantagefamily.com** or call **1.866.775.1696**.

To Mom and Dad, who gave me direction.
To my brother Danny, who always keeps me motivated.
To my children, who keep me humble.
And to my wife, Peggy, who keeps me balanced.

CONTENTS

FOREWORD XI

INTRODUCTION 1

CHAPTER 1
FINDING THE SOURCE 7

CHAPTER 2
PERIPHERAL NERVE INTEGRITY, JOINT ALIGNMENT, AND BALANCE 23

CHAPTER 3
BACK PAIN, BALANCE, BREATHING, AND STRENGTH—
A STRONG CONNECTION 51

CHAPTER 4
A LEVEL PELVIS—THE KEY TO CORE STABILITY AND BALANCE 67

CHAPTER 5
BETTER JOINTS, FEWER REPLACEMENT SURGERIES 77

CHAPTER 6
BETTER BONES, BETTER OVERALL HEALTH 91

CHAPTER 7
NONSURGICAL TREATMENTS FOR SPORTS AND OTHER INJURIES 109

CHAPTER 8
SURGERY—WHEN IT'S RIGHT 123

CONCLUSION
MAKING THE CORRECT DIAGNOSIS IS MOST IMPORTANT 143

APPENDIX 147

OUR PILLARS OF SERVICE 157

FOREWORD

"Reputation is what men and
women think of us; character is what
God and angels know of us."
THOMAS PAINE

have devoted most of my professional life to helping people with chronic face and head pain. Most of our treatments in the early days were centered around pain management. We helped in traditional ways to give some symptomatic (short term) relief with various therapies, though we understood the patient would have these ailments for the rest of their life. It was quite defeating to see the same patients week after week never healing fully or resolved of their problems—until I focused on the origin of their pain.

After years of training, education and research, I was finding success with a delivery model centered around breathing and the origin of pain. We heal when we sleep, so it was clear that breathing had a major impact on the chronically ill.

I have been teaching these techniques to specifically dentists for many years, throughout the world, and it is through these teachings I came to meet a very special man, orthopaedic surgeon Dr. Victor "Rocky" Romano.

An orthopaedic surgeon is at the top of the food chain when it comes to the physical and structural problems people suffer from. I was anxious to meet such a man who was so accomplished and competent in his knowledge and technique, yet so open to possibly learn from a dentist about orthopaedic injury.

Dr. Romano is the ultimate "doctor"—always searching for knowledge to improve the quality of life for others. His passion is abundant and infectious. Professionally, he teaches us all how to be the best we can be and to always think of the patient first. Personally, he is a role model for life, with the perfect balance and emphasis on family and career.

I know you will enjoy this book as much as I have. It is a series of explanations highlighted by examples of patients who had these problems. If you or someone you know suffer from chronic orthopaedic pain and you are trying to find answers, this book is for you. You will see yourself or the person you care for in the patients he describes. He will give you answers and help you make some tough decisions.

That is his mission in life. He is a man of character.

Sincerely,
Steven R. Olmos, D.D.S.
Board Certified in Craniofacial Pain
Board Certified in Dental Sleep Medicine
Founder of TMJ & Sleep Therapy Centres International

INTRODUCTION

From as early as I can remember, I knew I was going to be a doctor. I was named after my maternal grandfather, Vito Antonio Desolato Taglia, an old-time family physician who specialized in tuberculosis. All the other men in my family—my paternal grandfather, my father, my brothers, my uncle, and my cousin—were all in the wholesale liquor business. That really left no room for me in the family business, so I was going to be a doctor like my namesake—and that was that.

Since I needed good grades to be a doctor, I studied hard and became valedictorian at Fenwick High School. I was also a Tony Lawless Scholar Athlete my senior year in football and track. At five-foot-five and 125 pounds, I wasn't the greatest of athletes. I played wide receiver my senior year and never caught a pass in a year that ended 0–9. I still have occasional neck and back pain from play in my sophomore year when I was the varsity football wedge-buster. That meant my job was to dive headlong into a wedge created by three 200-plus-pound players on the opposing team. It was a suicide mission every time and is no longer allowed in football.

At the University of Notre Dame, I participated in boxing and rugby, and ultimately graduated cum laude in microbiology. Near the end of my junior year, when *Sports World* listened in my corner during my championship lightweight fight on national TV after I had been hit a few times, all I was able to mumble was "more salt," referring to smelling salts that were used to aid dazed competitors. Later, I underwent nasal surgery to fix all the years of damage from being an athlete, and my ear, nose, and throat (ENT) doctor remarked, "You didn't block many punches, did you?" These experiences have made me extremely diligent in protecting athletes with head injuries.

Though I was destined to be a doctor, and my mother was a doctor's daughter, I rarely went to a physician as a child. My mom believed doctor visits spelled trouble. "The doctor only finds things wrong with you. If you don't take a temperature, you don't have a fever," she always said.

By the time I got to college, I was still unsure whether I was going to be a doctor because it was right for me or because it would please my parents. My dad's answer was, "If you want to be a doctor to please me, then please me."

Finally, to help me feel better about the decision to pursue medicine, I spent a couple of summers in Vermont with my cousin, who was a family physician. That's when I finally knew medicine was for me. Later, I would discover those summers were the fun part of medicine. I wasn't exposed to the long hours of studying, being on call, the routine forty-hour shifts, and the middle-of-the-night emergencies. But that's all part of a career I enjoy immensely.

My formal medical training came from Loyola Stritch School of Medicine, where I was exposed to several different specializations, starting with cardiology, then cardiac surgery, then pediatrics. Of them all, I loved surgery the most because it gave me the chance to help people quickly. Unlike family or internal medicine, where a patient was administered medication and had to wait to see whether or not it worked, surgery gave immediate gratification.

My residency began in general surgery at Loyola University.

Although I was busy and loved to operate, I realized I wasn't truly happy—even after lengthy surgeries, too often people still died.

Thankfully, I was fortunate enough to do a three-month rotation in orthopaedic surgery just as the medical center was becoming a trauma center. The center was incredibly busy; when I wasn't on call, I was coming home late. I rarely saw my family, but I loved the work I was doing—helping otherwise-healthy people who had suffered major trauma. We did extensive surgeries, and afterward, the patients healed and were back on their feet. That's when I switched to the orthopaedic residency program at Loyola, where I did one year of research and five more years of orthopaedic surgery. My residency included six months at the University of Wisconsin in Madison and another three months at the University of Notre Dame doing orthopaedic sports medicine.

When I left my residency, I had two options—join a big group or go into private practice. The group I considered joining already had seven members, and is now a forty-person group. When I interviewed there, the founding partners placed a lot of emphasis on how much was billed every year. I then interviewed with Dr. Joseph Sheehan, an independent orthopaedist and my eventual partner, whose philosophy was simple: "Just do what's right." Private practice seemed to be a better fit for me.

We had an extraordinary Irish-Italian partnership for about twenty years until he retired. After that, I joined a twenty-seven-partner group and stayed with it for four years. When the group wanted to move my office a half hour away, I decided to stay in my hometown and continue with my own practice, Romano Orthopaedic Center. We are a neighborhood practice located in a near-west suburb of Chicago. My home is one block from where I grew up, and my practice is less than three miles from home.

I can honestly say I have been having the most fun I've ever had practicing medicine. Most recently, I've been joined by an outstanding young orthopaedist, Peter McQueen, MD, who completed his sports medicine fellowship in San Diego. My daughter, Maria Romano McGann, DO, is scheduled to join the practice upon completion of her foot and ankle surgery fellowship in Columbus, Ohio, in the summer of 2018. My son, Joe, is in his fourth year of medical school and is actively pursuing an orthopaedic residency with the intent of joining Romano Orthopaedics sometime during 2024.

Over the last twenty-five years, the most humbling experience I had in medicine was volunteering in Haiti one week after the devastating 2010 earthquake. Getting there after the earthquake was quite a challenge, but what greeted me and my companions in Port-au-Prince, the epicenter of the quake, was almost overwhelming: hundreds of people had been sitting, standing, or lying for days in a large open room, just waiting for help. Everyone we spoke to had the same story—the roof of their home had collapsed on them.

On our first day, my physician assistant and I placed dozens of children with broken femurs into body casts. After that, and until early in the morning, we took our turns performing amputations— with no medical attention for days, many people had no choice but to lose a limb. At five o'clock the next morning, a 6.5 aftershock shook the hospital, like a freight train was passing through next door. Amid the chaos and screams of all those terrified patients, we managed to get everyone outside to safety.

The injured kept on coming. Scores of people with crushed limbs and shattered dreams kept coming to the door, day after day. Yet all of them were very polite and thankful for what little we did for them. With few resources and a lot of hard work and ingenuity, we treated open wounds, fixed broken bones, and amputated what couldn't be saved. That is why I became a doctor—to help people in need. The hardest thing I had to do in Haiti was leave.

Today, patients come to me with pain in their neck, back, shoulder, hip, or knee and want a quick fix. But the body is very efficient when it comes to protecting itself against injury—so efficient, in fact, their pain may be a result of their body compensating for an injury elsewhere, far away from the presenting complaint. That's why I have evolved my orthopaedic surgery practice into one that finds the *source* of an injury, a process which includes both surgical and nonsurgical treatment options.

I wrote this book to help you better understand that, in order to heal completely, you must first find and treat the source of your problem.

This book is for readers of all ages and activity levels. It is for athletes who relentlessly work to be the best in their sport and don't want to lose all of their hard-earned accomplishments because of a debilitating injury that simply could have been avoided—no matter what anyone says. In the pages ahead, I will share how not only athletes but anyone can improve their balance to avoid injuries.

This book is also for everyday people who work hard from nine to five and try to stay in shape but have nagging injuries that keep them from working out regularly. If you're someone who avoids orthopaedic surgeons because you think all they do is operate, then read on. You'll see there are other options to consider that may help you avoid surgery—for the long term, or even altogether. In the pages ahead, you'll see how it's possible to find the source of your pain. I'll even share some simple techniques I teach my patients to help them reverse their injuries, allowing their bodies to heal on their own and keep them moving toward their goal of staying in shape without surgery.

This book also is written for those of you who are getting older and are at a greater risk of falling. You are one misstep away from breaking a bone and losing your independence. In the pages ahead, I will explain techniques to improve your balance and strengthen your bones.

Finally, this book is for those of you who have an injury that requires orthopaedic surgery. For you, looking for the source of your injury will help you recover more rapidly and completely from surgery and avoid future problems.

There are definitely times when orthopaedic surgery is the best solution. But in my practice, I'm not in a hurry to operate. We look to see whether there are nonsurgical options that should be considered first. Baseball Hall of Famer Satchel Paige said it best: "Don't run unless you're being chased." Don't run into surgery if you don't have to do so.

CHAPTER 1

FINDING THE SOURCE

E very time a patient comes to see me at my practice, I keep one thing at the top of my mind: The person in front of me is more than a hip or a knee or a shoulder in need of care. They are someone's mother, father, brother, or sister with a problem. That problem is affecting their lifestyle—not allowing that person to go out dancing at night or stand all day at work or exercise and play sports.

That's why I approach my practice as more than simply orthopaedic surgery. Yes, surgery is often the best solution for a health issue or injury. But at my practice, I believe in first finding the source of the problem. Finding the source means I don't just hurry to operate on the injury or issue at hand; I take the extra time to find and, whenever possible, treat the source of the problem with nonsurgical options. If I can help a patient get better without surgery, that's for the best.

Because I follow a philosophy of "finding the source," I have sometimes been referred to as an orthopaedic surgeon who doesn't like to operate. That's absolutely not true. I love to operate, and frankly, I'm very good at it. In fact, I have plenty of surgeries on my roster—as I write this chapter on a Sunday morning, I've just come out of my third surgery for a hip fracture this weekend. But I don't give away "frequent flyer miles" for surgery—the last thing I want is for a patient to have to keep returning to me for more and more surgery, which can happen with some conditions.

While I love what I do, I also love coming home for dinner and spending quality time with my wife, children, and grandchildren. So, if you need surgery, you can bet you will get extraordinary care from me. And if you can get better without surgery, all the better.

What it all comes down to is peeling back the layers to figure out what is contributing to your pain, what might prevent your pain from returning, or what can be done to improve your outcomes, whatever the treatment plan. Over the years, I've learned that if I want someone to heal completely and not come back for another surgery, it's critical to get to the source of the problem first.

For instance, when seventy-eight-year-old Bella fell in the bathroom and ended up in the emergency room, I fixed her hip the following morning—but that was far from my last interaction with her. I checked her for osteoporosis and set her up with a medical and nutritional program to strengthen her bones. I also diagnosed problems she was having with her feet and hands, which were throwing off her balance. I showed her how to correct those problems herself, so she could continually improve her balance. I also discovered she had sleep apnea (chronic breathing disruptions during sleep), which is what sent her to the bathroom in the middle of the night. She didn't want to wear a CPAP machine, so I set her up with a specialist who made her an oral appliance. She now sleeps well throughout the night.

Or take Mary, a forty-year-old accountant who tripped on a curb and broke her right ankle, which is what brought her to my door. After the surgery, she still had lower back pain and vague left leg pain that had been bothering her for months, and therapy didn't help. Further examination revealed her lower back pain was related to obstructed breathing—she had broken her nose falling off a horse as a kid, and now, as an adult, that injury was still plaguing many other areas of her body. By simply applying a nasal strip, her back pain improved significantly, and after showing her an easy way to manipulate her left foot, her leg pain went away immediately. I also found that her vitamin D levels were way below normal, so she added dairy to her diet and began taking a daily vitamin D supplement. "I'm glad I broke my ankle and found you," Mary told me.

And then there was Chris, who came in with pain in his right shoulder after sliding into home base during a baseball game. He came in expecting an MRI of his shoulder and was thinking of scheduling his surgery late in the fall. But he was shocked when he left my office with no pain after a quick manipulation of his ribs. He went right back to playing ball but he doesn't slide any more (or so he says).

Finding and treating the source of an injury helps determine whether surgery is really warranted at that time. When surgery is recommended, it's still crucial to find the source to help improve surgical outcomes—in other words, to keep you from coming back for the same surgery again.

So again, there's a time and place for surgery. I perform surgery when it needs to be done. Until then, I know there are other ways to address health issues. I've built my practice and my reputation around being able to fix the presenting problem expeditiously and with excellent clinical skills.

MEDICINE IS AN ART

There is an old saying in surgery: "There is nothing that we can't make worse." With modern techniques, surgical care is always improving. These days, 90 to 95 percent of surgeries are successful. Still, that leaves a small percentage of surgeries that experience complications.

Universally, the chance of getting an infection, for instance, may be less than 1 percent—but again, there's still a chance. And the risk of complications is even higher for people with diabetes, heart disease, or other medical conditions. So, there are no guarantees when it comes to surgery. As a colleague of mine once put it, "If you want a guarantee, go to Sears." If a complication does arise (heaven forbid), I would rather have a patient say, "I had no choice. I needed the surgery," than to have him or her say, "I wish I never had that surgery."

Medicine is an art, not a science. My art is to make an accurate diagnosis and teach you how to help yourself. I will also send you to our therapists, who understand that everything is connected—they can follow those connections and often get to the source of your problem. If therapy or other resources we have at our disposal don't fix the problem and make you feel better—ideally, pain-free—then surgery is likely your best option.

When it comes to finding the source, what intrigues me even more is finding out why and how you got to where you are. Hippocrates, the father of medicine, said, "Illnesses do not come upon us out of the blue. They are developed from small daily sins against Nature. When enough sins have accumulated, illnesses will suddenly appear." He was talking about how an injury to the body will manifest itself in pain elsewhere. I'll talk about this more in the chapters ahead, but that's what I see often in my practice, and that's why I've found that getting to the source is critical.

I WAS A SKEPTIC

I discovered the "finding the source" approach I now use today in my orthopaedic practice at a family Christmas party. My nephew, Dr. Daniel Klauer, a dentist specializing in the temporomandibular joint (TMJ) and sleep disordered breathing, was conducting a "medical show" in the hallway. He was testing everyone's balance and performing some strange maneuvers that I had never seen before. He would then tell his hallway "patients" the source of their pain—a foot, lower back, neck, or wherever. After he was finished with them, they came to me one by one. I examined the area he said was causing them pain, only to find nothing wrong. "He's a dentist," I said. "What does he know?"

Both intrigued and skeptical of what he was doing, I spoke to Daniel about this new technique and was surprised when he explained that it was developed by an orthopaedic surgeon, Dr. John Beck, and published in a non–peer-reviewed journal in 2008. The journal articles, titled "Practical Application of Neuropostural Evaluations" and "Neurobiological Basis for Chronic Pain," discussed the multilevel method of diagnosing patients with chronic pain.[1]

Daniel's mentor, Dr. Steven Olmos, also a dentist, had seen Dr. Beck present his new technique of balance and reflex testing at a pain conference and recognized it as a game changer. Dr. Olmos shadowed Dr. Beck once a week for a year and then used what he learned to develop a course for dentists. Dr. Beck's technique proved to be useful in treating patients with temporomandibular disorders (TMD), a condition that causes pain in the jaw. For instance, if a patient had TMD, he or she also would have one of Dr. Beck's described reflexes specific for TMD. Dr. Olmos then would make an oral appliance (a mouth guard) to alleviate his or her pain. If the reflex went away while wearing the appliance, Dr. Olmos knew treatment with that

---

1   JL Beck, "Neurodevelopmental Basis for Chronic Regional Pain Syndrome," *Practical Pain Management* 8, no. 6 (2008): 44–53, https://www.practicalpainmanagement.com/pain/neuropathic/crps/neurodevelopmental-basis-chronic-regional-pain-syndrome; "Practical Application of Neuropostural Evaluations," *Practical Pain Management* 8, no. 7 (2008): 47–53, https://www.practicalpainmanagement.com/resources/diagnostic-tests/practical-application-neuropostural-evaluations

appliance would work. If the reflex did not go away while wearing the appliance, he would have to try another solution.

After the holiday gathering, Daniel enthusiastically persuaded me to learn the technique. He called my wife, blocked my office schedule and booked my flight. Reluctantly, I agreed, and off I went to the conference in Toronto.

Before the conference began, Daniel told me he thought his business partner had torn his rotator cuff and asked me to examine him. In my initial examination, I found he had good strength in his rotator cuff muscles, pain in his shoulder when twisting his neck, and weakness in straightening his elbow.

"It's not his rotator cuff," I concluded. "It's coming from his neck." I was convinced his pain was coming from his C7 nerve root, something every orthopaedist would know.

Then, Dr. Olmos examined him and agreed the problem was not his rotator cuff—but he said it was coming from his lower back, on the opposite side from the pain.

"That's it!" I thought. "I'm going home. Who is this crazy dentist, telling me, an orthopaedic surgeon, that it's not his neck but coming from his lower back? I'm wasting my time here." Unable to really escape the situation, I sat in the back of the classroom, completely disinterested.

Dr. Olmos began the conference by telling attendees how Dr. Beck observed that patients who experienced certain orthopaedic injuries often resorted back to the infant reflexes that normally disappear during early childhood. Dr. Beck also observed patients who had these reflexes also experienced a loss in balance. Then Dr. Olmos started talking about TMD. As an orthopaedist, I operate on important joints like the hip and the knee. I didn't care about the jaw—that wasn't my realm.

Amid my disinterest, I heard Dr. Olmos mention that TMD is five to eight times more common in girls than in boys. Suddenly, a light bulb went on. I sat up and started paying attention. Why? Because I knew in noncontact sports, anterior cruciate ligament (ACL) tears (in the knee) are five to eight times more common in girls than in boys—the same rate of incidence as TMD. As every sports medicine specialist knows, girls have less balance than boys.[2] Studies have shown that if girls undergo a special balance program for several weeks, their ACL tear rate is lessened to roughly the same rate as boys. "Could it be that girls with TMD are the same ones tearing their ACLs?" I wondered. "If that were the case, all I would need to do would be to give them a mouth guard to improve their balance and lower their rate of ACL tears. Could it really be that simple?"

The conference involved demonstrating the reflexes one at a time and participants trying the reflex tests on each other. I was the only orthopaedist in a group of twenty-two dentists. On the last day, we were finally going to test the lower back. I couldn't wait to prove Dr. Olmos wrong about his diagnosis of my nephew's business partner.

Sure enough, the test showed his problem was coming from his lower back on the opposite side. I asked for some lidocaine to inject into his lower back, which, if ineffective, would prove my point—that his pain was coming from his neck, not his lower back. But when I injected his lower back, not only did his shoulder pain go away but his strength also returned to normal. I was dumbfounded. All my years of training seemed to be turned upside down.

---

2 Natalie Voskanian, "ACL Injury prevention in female athletes: review of the literature and practical consideration sin implementing an ACL prevention program," *Current Reviews in Musculoskeletal Medicine* 6, no. 2 (June 2013)158–163, https://doi.org/10.1007/s12178-013-9158-y

A NEW DIRECTION

I returned home with an anxious enthusiasm to test my patients. The first patient I saw was Cristina, who was recently in a automobile accident. She told me she was miserable because severe neck pain was keeping her up at night. She asked for a cortisone injection in her neck to relieve her pain. Instead, I told her about the course I just had completed, and asked if she would let me try my new reflex testing on her. She agreed. It turned out from my tests that the source of her pain was the opposite lower back, too. It took some convincing before she would let me give her an injection in her lower back for neck pain. But when I did, sure enough, the pain in her neck went away.

These days, I see similar problems routinely, and yet I'm still amazed each time I discover the source of the pain is coming from somewhere else in the body. It is now standard procedure for me to use Autonomic Motor Nerve Reflex Testing (AMNRT) on every patient, and I've developed a treatment program that lasts longer than the temporary relief of an injection—manipulating and strengthening the lower back and extremities. I will discuss AMNRT in depth in the next chapter.

Once I understood the body compensates for injuries—for instance, a patient may have shoulder pain because they are adapting their stance to accommodate a back injury—my orthopaedic practice entered a whole new world. Patients who come to me with problems leave feeling better right away.

Before my new direction, I often diagnosed their problem— tennis elbow, rotator cuff tendinitis, carpal tunnel syndrome (CTS), or something else—and sent them off to physical therapy, hoping for the best. If they didn't respond to therapy, I'd see them again, give them an injection, and again, hope for the best. If the injection didn't help, then surgery was often the next step. Most of the time, patients got better after surgery, but as you can imagine, it was a much longer process that involved taking time off work, missing out on sports, or putting their life on hold while they suffered in pain. And for some, even after surgery, a bit of nagging pain remained. That was a true source of frustration. Now that I treat the source of the pain instead of targeting only the location of the symptoms, patients are getting lasting relief much faster, sometimes without surgery.

For instance, before I began looking for the source of pain, I performed a knee arthroscopy on my friend, Sue, a fifty-five-year-old entrepreneur. Arthroscopy is a procedure using a small camera to look into the joint for diagnosis and treatment. In this case, I treated Sue's knee for a meniscus tear. She felt better after surgery, but after a few months, she was back with pain in the same knee. I diagnosed she needed more therapy, which included stretching and strengthening her hamstrings. The therapy eventually worked, but she came back a third time—this time after I had evolved the direction of my practice. She insisted she needed another surgery on her knee. With AMNRT testing, I found the source of her problem was coming from her opposite foot. She was having pain in the opposite foot so she was subconsciously putting more weight on her operative knee, causing pain.

"No, my foot doesn't hurt," she insisted.

But when I pressed between her toes on that foot, she nearly jumped off the exam table. The solution at the time was a toe spacer, but today, I have a program of manipulations and stretches that provide even longer-term relief.

She said, "It can't be that easy." It was. Her knee pain went away.

The evolution of my revamped practice wasn't easy. Although patients were getting better quickly and more completely, I found some colleagues and therapists thought I had gone a little crazy. In looking for the source, I often collaborate with professionals in other areas of medicine—dentistry, ENT, sleep specialists, nutritionists, therapists, and chiropractors. At first, I had some difficulty convincing a few of those other professionals that I needed them to provide treatment for patients in areas on their body other than where they were reporting symptoms. Because I am a surgeon, they expect me to target the area where the symptoms are occurring; they couldn't understand why I would point to somewhere else on the body as the source of a problem.

When I diagnosed Ruby, a middle-aged woman with shoulder pain, as needing therapy on her back as well as her shoulder, I brought the therapist I had been using for years into the treatment room to demonstrate how stretching the patient's lower back on the opposite side improved her shoulder pain, strength, and range of motion. The therapist wasn't convinced.

She refused to work on Ruby's back, saying, "It is unethical to work on the lower back for shoulder pain when the back doesn't hurt." I ended up finding a new physical therapist.

Another patient, Max, a forty-five-year-old security guard, had surgery for patellar tendinitis (in his knee). Postoperative physical therapy only worsened his symptoms. Finally, I diagnosed him with complex regional pain syndrome, a condition where the pain is out of proportion to the physical findings. In other words, his nerves were hyperactive—increasing his heart rate, constricting the blood vessels, and causing his pain to go out of control. Only medical marijuana provided him relief, and after second and third opinions, he was placed on total disability. But after I evolved my practice to finding the source, I discovered Max had sleep apnea and needed nasal surgery to clear his obstructed breathing.

When I told a pulmonary colleague about Max's turnaround now that he was able to breathe better, my colleague said, "They all get better with relaxation techniques," then turned and walked away. Today, Max is no longer on disability, no longer uses medical marijuana, and works full-time as a security guard.

Characterized by chronic muscle pain, fatigue, sleep problems, and painful trigger points, fibromyalgia is another diagnosis orthopaedic surgeons don't like to treat and, frankly, tend to avoid. There are no physical findings or diagnostic tests for fibromyalgia. There is no cure. Medication, exercise, relaxation, and stress-reduction measures can only help control symptoms. Surgery can make it worse. Although fibromyalgia patients aren't good surgical candidates, I enjoy the challenge of taking care of them. Almost every AMNRT reflex is positive on fibromyalgia patients, so using it can, for the first time, diagnose them with actual problems. Most patients have some combination of carpal and cubital tunnel syndromes, rib subluxation, TMD, and obstructed breathing with associated neck and back pain and sleep disturbance. Each problem needs to be addressed systematically, one at a time, so healing can finally begin.

I have had several physicians tell me I shouldn't be diagnosing sleep apnea: "That's not in your field!" When Jackson, a young, obese boy came to me with knee pain, I diagnosed the source as his lower back. But that back problem, I determined, was the result of obstructed breathing, which can result in sleep apnea. Jackson's mom reported he snored, which meant he needed a sleep study; the American Pediatric Society recommends a sleep study for any child who snores.[3]

---

3   Carole L. Marcus et al., "Diagnosis and Management of Childhood Obstructive Sleep Apnea Syndrome," *American Academy of Pediatrics* 130, no. 3 (August 2012): e714-55, https://doi.org/10.1542/peds.2012-1672

His pediatrician was annoyed with my suggestion of sleep apnea and said, "Tell him to go outside, run around, and play. That's all he needs." This saddened me greatly, as the doctor didn't send Jackson back to me to follow up.

When I shared this and other stories with my dental associates from the conference, they replied, "Welcome to my world!" In spite of some resistance from colleagues and therapists, my practice continues to grow because my patients are getting better.

PAIN IS SUBJECTIVE

So, while I'm an orthopaedic surgeon, I know too often patients are sent for surgery before other options are considered. Once the surgery is done, if it does not solve the problem, there are usually few other options left for the patient. The bottom line is that pain is subjective—people experience pain differently. One patient may rate their pain as a three out of ten, but similar pain may be rated as a nine by a different patient. One study found the more comorbidities (having two or more diseases or conditions at the same time), the more pain the patient may have—in other words, pain in one area may make them more susceptible to pain in another area.[4] For instance, the size of a rotator cuff tear may not correlate with the amount of pain a person is experiencing.[5] Their pain may be heightened by an injury from somewhere else in their body, and it's my job to find those comorbidities. If I can find and treat the source, then the area where a patient is experiencing pain may improve without the need for surgery.

---

4   Jessica Davis, et al., "Incidence and impact of pain conditions and comorbid illnesses," *Journal of Pain Research* 4 (October 2011): 331–345, https://doi.org/10.2147/JPR.S24170.

5   Dunn WR et al., "Symptoms of pain do not correlate with rotator cuff tear severity," *Journal of Bone and Joint Surgery* 96, no. 10 (May 21): 793–800, https://doi.org/10.2106/JBJS.L.01304

A review of orthopaedic studies found there was no correlation between the integrity of the repair and the outcome of surgery. The review looked at MRIs in patients who had rotator cuff repairs and found that 13 to 50 percent of those patients had recurrent rotator cuff tears after surgery. However, 80 to 90 percent of the patients had good to excellent results after surgery, with significant improvement whether or not they had a recurrent tear.[6] In other words, a person may have improved pain and function after an "unsuccessful" rotator cuff surgery or have persistent pain and weakness after a "successful" surgery. That's why it's important to find and treat the source of pain before surgery.

Carpal tunnel syndrome (CTS) can be particularly subjective. Patients with this condition often continue to experience pain and weakness after surgery. The literature often blames the pain on depression; as surgeons, we're advised not to perform carpal tunnel surgery on someone who is depressed.[7] I believe it's the other way around—if your hand is numb and hurts, making it hard to use it, you might get depressed at some point. I used to perform a lot of carpal tunnel surgeries, but today they are rarer—yet I'm seeing more patients with the condition. Why? Because I'm getting them better without surgery.

While I don't perform back surgeries in my practice, I successfully treat a lot of patients with back pain. Although necessary at times, surgery should be the last resort for back pain. As my chiro-

---

6   Russell RD et al., "Structural integrity after rotator cuff repair does not correlate with patient function and pain: a meta analysis," *Journal of Bone and Joint Surgery* 96, no. 4 (February 19): 265–271, https://doi.org/10.2106/JBJS.M.00265.

7   Jin Woo Park, "The Effect of Psychological Factors on the Outcomes of Carpal Tunnel Release: A Systematic Review," *Journal of Hand Surgery (Asian-Pacific Volume)* 22, no. 2 (June 2017): 131–137, https://doi.org/10.1142/S0218810417300029.

practor colleague says, "That's why they call it back surgery—because they always keep coming back for more surgery."

FINDING RELIEF

Today, my practice is more fun because people routinely are shocked when I discover the true source of their pain. After I reverse the process with a few simple techniques they can do themselves, they often leave my office in little or no pain. I've now begun to gather data to help measure the effectiveness of my techniques, which may lead to even more exciting changes as I continue to evolve my practice.

My goal is to help everyone relieve their pain, whether through tried-and-true nonsurgical options or through surgery, should it be needed. I don't want anyone to endure pain when there are so many options to alleviate it. Just look at some of the pro athletes today whose careers are struggling because they can't seem to find the source of their pain, or because they're trying options that simply don't work—Tiger Woods and Derrick Rose are just a couple of the big names that come to mind.

But in my practice, I'm continually working with athletes of all ages who are finding relief from aggravating injuries that have interfered with their career. For instance, an all-pro running back who had multiple injuries during his career had returned to play after reconstructive knee surgery, only to retire a short time later with chronic lower back pain. Many years afterwards, he came to see me. I found that manipulating his foot and giving him a breathing strip to wear on his nose helped him regain both his strength and his balance. "I wish I knew this back then," he told me.

My point is that you're going to keep on getting hurt unless you fix the source of the problem. No matter how hard you work, no matter how good you are at what you do, you can still end up with problems if you have poor balance because of some other injury of which you may not even be aware. In fact, I've found balance is so important that it's the first thing I look for in every new patient. I will discuss this in more detail in the next three chapters.

CHAPTER 2

PERIPHERAL NERVE INTEGRITY, JOINT ALIGNMENT, AND BALANCE

K yle, a twenty-three-year-old, rookie professional football player, recently had been cut by the New Orleans Saints. Thirty minutes before the Chicago Bears called him for an evaluation and possible signing, he broke his left foot while running a pass pattern. It was not an ordinary foot fracture but a Jones fracture. Whenever a fracture gets a special name, you know it's a problem fracture. Since Jones fractures are at the base of the fifth metatarsal (midfoot) where the blood supply is poor, they are slow to heal. Surgical correction is a good idea, especially in an athlete who wants to return to sports quickly.

Kyle had already suffered a Jones fracture in his right foot during his sophomore year in college. He had a successful surgical correction and returned to play in full force his junior year. Even though he caught the winning pass that beat Notre Dame at the end of his senior year, I forgave him (for beating my team) and scheduled his surgery on his left foot the following day.

An outstanding athlete, Kyle was in extraordinary shape. However, when I tested him using AMNRT, he lost his balance when

23

he closed his eyes or stared at my black suit. With AMNRT, I found that he actually had unambiguous tenderness in his right foot—but he had no idea that he had a problem in that area. The injury to his left foot most likely occurred because his body was subconsciously compensating to protect the injured right foot. That caused him to lose his balance while running and making a sharp cut, which led to the left foot fracture. After I manipulated his right foot, the patho-logic reflex—that subconscious compensation factor—disappeared, and his balance improved immediately. Too bad he hadn't known that before practicing that day.

BALANCE—THE KEY TO GOOD HEALTH

When patients present me with problems, balance is the first thing I look for using AMNRT reflex testing, an exceptional tool I have in my orthopaedic diagnostic tool kit. As an orthopaedic surgeon, I am expertly trained to treat a wide range of injuries with many different courses of treatment. But unfortunately, it's common practice for orthopaedic surgeons as a whole to focus on patient complaints, physical findings, X-rays, and MRIs to make the diagnosis. The use of AMNRT reflex testing allows me to go beyond conventional teachings and find the true source of an injury.

The human body is adeptly designed to compensate for injuries. That's why at times, as in Kyle's case, the presenting complaint may be some place on the body far removed from the underly-ing source of the injury. Although surgical correction of the Jones fracture was Kyle's best option, quickly finding and correcting the true source of the problem significantly improved his postoperative rehabilitation and decreased his chances of having another noncon-tact injury when he returned to football.

Balance in life is important—balance between work and play, activity and rest. You can't just work out all day long. You have to let the body heal itself. You can't just study all day long. You need to rest your mind.

Balance is also the key to good health. When your body is out of balance, you will begin to experience a myriad of problems. A loss of balance indicates something is wrong internally. It's a clue to look further.

I use a systematic balance assessment to diagnose the health of the following three neuromuscular systems:

- **The peripheral nervous system**, which involves the nerves to the hands, feet, elbows, ribs, jaw, and pelvis. If your peripheral nervous system is off, then your balance will be off when you close your eyes or look at a dark color. I will discuss this system later in this chapter.

- **The central nervous system**, which involves the nerves to the neck and back and is also associated with nasal breathing. If your breathing is off, then you will have problems with your back. If you lose your balance when you turn your head to the left or right, or nod your head up and down, then your central nervous system is off. I will discuss this more in chapter three.

- **Pelvic alignment.** If your pelvis is out of alignment, one side of your body will be weaker than the other. Normally, a big guy whose balance is fine could toss me like a ragdoll. But if his balance is off, he can easily be toppled over during a balance test. I also have found that if the pelvis is off, the shoulder will be tight. I will discuss this more in chapter four.

The protocol I'm going to share with you is what I use currently, but it is constantly evolving. While Dr. Beck described several reflexes to test nerves, I have found additional ones. The human body has many nerves, all of which may have their own reflexes that are yet to be discovered. That is what makes orthopaedic surgery still exciting to me after twenty-five years in practice.

AMNRT OF THE PERIPHERAL NERVES

The first in the series of tests I conduct is based on the initial reflex humans have as infants. It is known as the light/dark reflex. Simply put, when the lights are off, an infant goes to sleep. It's like a natural-born instinct, or reflex, for the infant body to shut down in the dark. That reflex is something everyone outgrows.

However, Dr. Beck discovered in adulthood, when the peripheral nervous system is in distress or, as he says, "in dystrophy," the body reverts to that primitive reflex of automatically shutting down in the dark. The peripheral nervous system includes the nerves to your hands, feet, elbows, ribs, jaw, and pelvis. These nerves tell your muscles what to do; your body's movements rely on your nervous system for instructions. When there is a problem in the system—when one of the peripheral nerves is irritated, whether or not you actually sense pain—the system that moves your body is disrupted, causing you to lose your strength and balance in the dark.

When testing patients for the light/dark reflex, I ask them to stand rigid, facing me, with their arms to their side and elbows flexed to 90 degrees. I ask patients to focus their eyes on me, and then I try to push them off-balance—their ability to remain rigid at that point gives me a baseline understanding. Then I ask them to close their eyes and try to remain rigid while I again try to push them off-balance. If they are able to keep their balance, then their peripheral nervous system is intact. If they lose their balance, they are in dystrophy.

Patients are usually amazed when I'm able to push them off-balance. Some call it voodoo, others call it magic. Some say I am pushing harder when they close their eyes, but I assure you I am not. I am not trying to fool anyone. It's simply the way the reflex works.

Sometimes during the test, patients are in such disbelief as to how it works they try to overpower me. I have to remind them this is a reflex test to check their balance so I can get to the source of their problem. It is not a strength test. Being only five foot five and 145 pounds, I don't want to get hurt in a shoving match when I'm trying to help someone understand how to resolve their pain. Although, I have to admit, I smile a little on the inside when I can knock a big, 250-pound man off-balance.

The light/dark reflex test, in addition to balance, also allows me to test a patient's strength with his or her eyes open and then with them closed. This is especially useful with patients who cannot stand: for instance, when they have an ankle fracture or a broken hip. Patients in dystrophy will have normal strength with their eyes open and lose their strength with their eyes closed.

When patients test light/dark positive, I repeat the test, but this time I ask them to stare at a dark object instead of me. When they again lose their balance and strength, they are even more perplexed. "How can that be?" they want to know. Again, it's simply a reflex. At least one of their peripheral nerves is irritated—possibly more. (Perhaps that's why teams who wear dark colors like red or black win more than teams who wear light colors[8]—unless Tom Brady is on your team.) After this test, I need to find out which peripheral nerve or nerves are irritated by conducting a series of scratch tests.

---

8   Russell A. Hill and Robert A. Barton, "Psychology: Red enhances human performance in contests," *Nature: International Journal of Science,* May 18, 2005, https://www.nature.com/articles/435293a

SCRATCH TESTS

If the light/dark test is positive, I take the patient through a series of scratch/withdrawal reflexes. Like the knee-jerk reflex—when the doctor sits you down and then taps you on the knee with a small hammer—scratch tests evaluate a collection of involuntary reflexes to determine the actual injured or irritated nerve or nerves causing the pathologic, or abnormal, withdrawal response.

Just as the AMNRT tests are based on an infantile reflex, so too are the scratch tests. Adults don't automatically react to someone lightly scratching on their skin, but infants do—they instinctively withdraw from it. That's why when babies are born, doctors don't slap them on their bottom to get them to cry, like you see in old movies; they scratch their feet. Similarly, patients whose bodies are in dystrophy will revert to that infantile reflex and withdraw from a scratch. If there is no dystrophy, then the patient won't withdraw when scratched—it's that simple.

The truly mystifying aspect of these reflexes is that the area scratched is usually nowhere near the irritated nerve. For instance, if someone scratches their right arm over the ulnar nerve and they withdraw, that means the problem may be stemming from their right foot—the plantar nerve in the right foot is irritated and is a precursor to Morton's neuroma. They will be tender over their right foot when I squeeze it. When they withdraw from a scratch on their left little finger, it means the median nerve in the right wrist is irritated. You can bet they will have weakness in their right thumb and tenderness over the median nerve in the right wrist when I push on it—all diagnostic of CTS. Don't ask, "Why?" It defies logic! I tell my patients, "I didn't hook us up. And the Big Guy who did, unfortunately, didn't leave us with any blueprints."

Patients may be unaware of their nerve injuries until I point it out to them. Often when I do so, the responses I get are, "It didn't hurt until you poked me!" or "I feel it, but it doesn't really hurt." Nerve pain may not hurt as much as bone or joint pain hurts. Nevertheless, the body still subconsciously feels the pain and compensates for it. Our brain doesn't care about pain, it cares about survival.

NERVE INJURIES AND REPAIR

Dr. John Beck has described eight reflexes associated with nerve injuries and various musculoskeletal entities, and in the four years I have used this diagnostic tool, I have found four additional reflexes. I am certain there are more to be found.

To confirm his findings when testing for the reflexes, Dr. Beck would inject the injured nerve with lidocaine. If the reflex went away and the pain improved, then that nerve was the source of the pain. But I'm most excited to report that instead of masking the pain and reflex with lidocaine injections, I can now reverse these pathologic reflexes and alleviate pain in many cases with mobilization and stretching of the affected areas.

There are several reflexes that can be affected and that help diagnose a problem. Let's look at some of the reflexes I see most commonly in my practice:

- Peroneal neuropathy
- Morton's neuroma
- CTS
- Cubital tunnel syndrome
- TMD
- Posterior rib subluxation
- Sports hernia

PERONEAL NEUROPATHY AND MORTON'S NEUROMA

Two reflexes I see commonly affect the feet: peroneal neuropathy and Morton's neuroma. The peroneal nerve ends on the top of the foot, between the first and second toes. When there is sensitivity of the peroneal nerve, it's most likely to be in the first web space—that stretch of skin between the base of the big and second toes. Morton's neuroma is the name given to an irritated plantar nerve branch, which ends on the bottom of the foot between the third and fourth toes. The most common symptoms of peroneal neuropathy of the foot and Morton's neuroma are burning pain, numbness, and/or tingling of toes and/or the ball of the foot. Most of the time, the pain is ignored or goes unnoticed until it is pointed out. Last year, when I tested our local university's men's soccer team (I am the team physician), 60 percent of our athletes had a positive foot reflex, yet no one complained of foot pain.

Even more common are patients with problems in their lower extremities, such as arthritis, ankle fractures, meniscus tears, muscle cramps, neuropathies, and plantar fasciitis, who also have compression of the peroneal nerves and/or Morton's neuromas in their feet—the true source of their pain. Usually, these lesions or injuries are on the opposite limbs of their problems.

For example, a sixty-five-year-old gentleman came to see me with pain in his right knee, and X-rays showed mild arthritis there. Upon examination, he had tenderness to palpation of his right knee, but with AMNRT I found tenderness over the peroneal nerve on his left foot. He didn't even realize it until I pointed it out. His mind ignored or even shut out the pain so he could keep on walking. However, his body still felt the pain and compensated for it. This subconsciously caused him to favor his left foot, putting more weight on his right leg while walking—in turn, making his right knee feel worse.

Alternately, because an irritated nerve automatically throws off your balance, you might easily lose your balance and tear the meniscus in your right knee or fracture your right hip or ankle while subconsciously protecting the left foot. With traditional orthopaedic care, the meniscus tear or the fracture would be fixed to get you back in the game as soon as possible—but then you would return with more injuries (think Derrick Rose.) Using AMNRT, I not only fix your presenting complaint but also take care of the underlying sources of your injury so you may return to your sport or daily activities safely, without any unnecessary fear of a recurrent injury.

The ankle is a natural shock absorber for the lower extremities when walking, running, lunging, or jumping. If your calf muscles are tight, your ankle doesn't dorsiflex (bend upward toward your knee) all the way to absorb the shock. Consequently, the ball of the foot takes a pounding, throwing your foot out of alignment and, thus, irritating the nearby nerves. Therefore, it is important to wear good, supportive shoes and stretch your ankles several times a day to stop this pathologic cycle and prevent recurrent injuries.

Reversing nerve irritation is important in healing. Without taking care of the source of an injury, you will not get better or you will return with a new injury. When your foot is out of alignment, the nearby nerves are irritated, causing dystrophy. I found that maximally plantarflexing your foot (bending your ankle so that your toes point away from your knee) will realign your foot, stop the irritation of the nerve, and restore your balance.

A while back, I was sitting at the nurses' station in between surgeries when a doctor asked me to consult on a patient with right knee pain. The patient was a seventy-five-year-old veteran in rehab because of marked weakness after a recent bout of pneumonia. In looking at his X-rays, I noted he had a fair amount of arthritis in his right knee. Since the patient was slowly making his way down the hallway with his walker—while a therapist held onto a gait belt around his waist and an orderly followed closely behind with a wheelchair in case the man grew tired and needed to rest—I performed an examination right there in the hallway. I sat the man in his wheelchair and knelt in front of him. Quickly testing his dark/light response and Morton's reflex, I said with a little bit of drama, "Obviously, it's coming from his left foot."

The man responded, "Yeah, I hurt my foot several weeks ago."

I then manipulated the man's foot and instructed him, "Get up and walk!"

The man stood up from the wheelchair, let go of his walker, and with no assistance from the therapist, walked straight back to his room. I headed back toward the operating room.

They're still talking about that today.

Foot Stretches to Reverse Peroneal Neuropathy and Morton's Neuroma Reflexes:

If your knees are good, kneel down and sit straight-up on your feet. In Japan, this is called *seiza*, the traditional, formal way of sitting. It is also an integral part of martial arts.

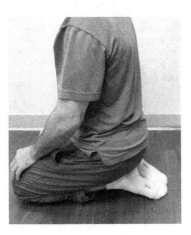

You also can stretch your foot with your hand. Alternatively, if your knee is bad, you can stretch your foot by standing and placing the top of your foot on the seat of a chair behind you (have something to hold on in front of you).

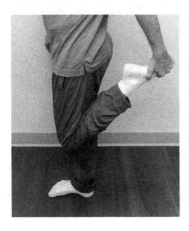
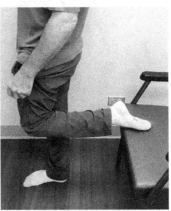

To stretch your right heel, bring your right leg back, keep the knee straight and foot flat on the ground. Lean against the wall with both hands, supporting yourself with your left leg. Hold the stretch for a slow count of three, for three reps. Then, repeat for the left heel.

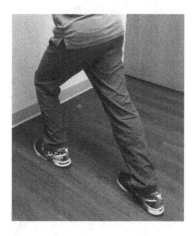

Do not hyper-extend your foot—where your toes point toward your knee. These pathologic foot reflexes may return by doing so and throw off your balance once again. Examples of these "don't do" stretches are standing wall calf stretches and calf raises.

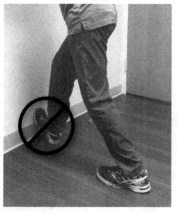 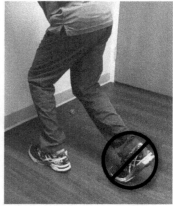

To avoid recurrence of injuries, wear shoes with good arch supports and always stretch your heels with both feet flat on the ground.

CARPAL TUNNEL SYNDROME

Carpal Tunnel Syndrome (CTS) is pain, numbness, and weakness of the hand caused by entrapment of the median nerve at the wrist. The carpal tunnel is the channel in the bones at your wrist through which the nerve travels. Patients usually associate their symptoms with waking up from sleep, holding a steering wheel or another object for a more extended period than normal, or prolonged use of the hand, such as while typing or working on an assembly line. Through AMNRT, I find that many patients with complaints in their upper extremities frequently have underlying CTS causing, or at least aggravating, their pain.

Diabetes, pregnancy, obesity, hypothyroidism, and heavy manual labor are some predisposing factors to CTS. I also have found that extreme dorsiflexion of the wrist (flexing the hand upward) while doing push-ups, burpees, improper weight lifting, or even pushing up to get out of a chair may throw the wrist out of alignment, irritating the median nerve and causing CTS. Such movements must be avoided.

Classically, treatment for CTS includes a wrist splint during heavy use of the affected arm and while sleeping, proper ergonomics at work, physical therapy, injections, and surgery—all with varying results. I have found that when the wrist is subluxed (out of alignment), the median nerve that runs through the carpal tunnel is aggravated, causing the familiar CTS symptoms. By reducing the subluxation through manipulation of the wrist, the irritation of the nerve is eliminated, and full strength and sensation are restored. Note: forcefully extending your wrist (pushing off your palms, like doing pushups) may take your wrist out of alignment and repeat this pathologic cycle.

Since learning the above information, I have significantly reduced the number of carpal tunnel surgeries I perform. Instead, I make many of my patients better by simply manipulating their wrists. I also teach them how to self-manipulate their own wrists and how to avoid recurring subluxations. Simply grab the back of your hand while resting your forearm on your belly. Now pull on your wrist and bend it downward. That's it! This will bring the wrist back into alignment, reverse the median nerve irritation, and relieve CTS symptoms. Frequent pulling of your wrist while avoiding forced extension will prevent CTS symptoms from recurring. While these treatments work for many patients, occasionally the damage from CTS is too severe, and surgery is necessary.

However, that wasn't the case with a forty-five-year-old police officer who came to see me for carpal tunnel surgery. He was off work for a couple of weeks with pain, weakness, and numbness of both hands—classic CTS. His wife had carpal tunnel surgery several years earlier and returned to work six weeks after surgery, so he wanted the same treatment. Instead, I manipulated his wrists, and most of his pain and tingling went away and his strength returned instantly. He was amazed that he could get back so much functionality without surgery. I had him temporarily wear a wrist brace and avoid dorsi-flexing his wrist. Within a couple of weeks, he returned to full-duty police work without surgery.

Using AMNRT, I have found CTS associated with vague pain in the shoulder, elbow, forearm, wrist, and/or hand, including rotator cuff tendinitis, tennis or golfer's elbow, De Quervain's syndrome (teno-synovitis of the wrist and thumb), and trigger finger. Reversing the carpal tunnel reflex significantly reduces these associated symptoms.

Stretches to Reverse the Carpal Tunnel Reflex:

To reduce wrist subluxation, perform the same stretch I mentioned earlier: grab the back of your hand while resting your forearm on your belly. Now simply pull on your wrist while bending it downward. You may or may not hear a "pop." Regardless, your pain and numbness should decrease, and your strength should return. Do this as often as necessary.

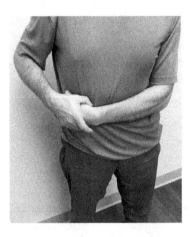

Always keep wrists straight when lifting and pushing.

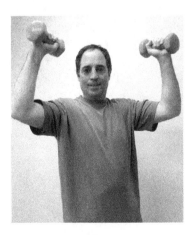

Do push-ups with weights, your fists, or the heels of your hands.

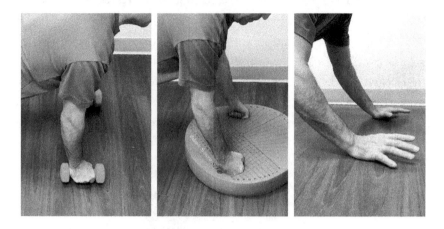

Always avoid extreme extension of the wrist when pushing and lifting.

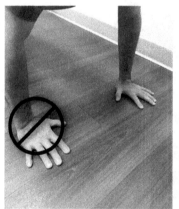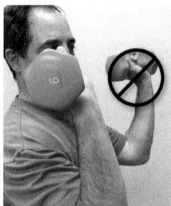

CUBITAL TUNNEL SYNDROME

Like CTS, cubital tunnel syndrome occurs because of a trapped nerve in the body—this time involving the ulnar nerve in the elbow. The ulnar nerve is your "funny bone." Have you ever bumped your elbow and felt brief but intense pain and numbness that radiates down to the ring and little fingers? That's because you bumped your ulnar nerve. The cubital tunnel is the channel in the bone at your elbow through which the nerve travels.

Treatment classically includes elbow splints for work and/or sleep, physical and occupational therapy, injections, and, if all else fails, surgery. Surgery, however, isn't always successful. I have found an easier, less-invasive treatment.

Like CTS, cubital tunnel syndrome is associated with subluxation—but at the elbow, not the wrist. When the elbow is subluxed, the ulnar nerve that runs behind the elbow is irritated, causing pain, numbness, weakness, and tingling that goes down to the ring and little fingers. Manipulating the elbow reverses the nerve irritation and restores the strength and sensation.

A common cause of elbow subluxation is rapid flexion of the elbow past 90 degrees in weightlifting and certain exercises.

Like CTS, cubital tunnel syndrome also is associated with vague pain in the shoulder, elbow, forearm, wrist, and/or hand and with pain caused by wrist or rotator cuff tendinitis and tennis or golfer's elbow. Reversing the cubital tunnel reflex also reduces these associated symptoms.

Melissa was a thirty-five-year-old bartender who told me she had pain in both wrists, which had been bothering her for several months. By the time she came to see me, she was on the verge of tears. The week before, she had gone to the ER where she was given pain medication that made her "loopy," as well as anti-inflammatory medicine that upset her stomach. Determined to find answers, she studied CTS online and then came to see me for surgical correction.

She had a classic case of CTS, so I could have scheduled her for surgery and moved on to my next patient. Instead, I checked her balance using AMNRT and found that she had both carpal and cubital tunnel syndromes. Manipulation of both wrists and elbows relieved a lot of her pain. I showed her how to do the manipulations herself and how to avoid aggravating her wrists and elbows during the day. I also gave her wrist braces to be worn at night.

Testing also revealed she had obstructed breathing with corresponding neck pain and shoulder weakness (see chapter three). She said the pain in those areas of her body was annoying but didn't stop her from working.

Then, I looked into her mouth and saw that her tongue was scalloped and her teeth were worn down. With questioning, I found that she woke up two to three times per night to use the bathroom, but she thought that was normal because she drank a lot of water. She also admitted she was a little tired during the day. "But isn't everybody?" she asked. She had seasonal allergies for which over-the-counter antihistamines gave little to no relief. I gave her a nasal strip, which instantly cleared her breathing, improved her strength, and decreased her pain. "Wow! I feel a rush," she said. "I didn't know I was supposed to breathe like that." That's when she smiled for the first time since entering my office.

Finally, I tested her core balance and found that her left side was off (see chapter four). "That's my weak side," she reported. After I showed her how to do a simple sacral stretch, her left side suddenly became stronger. The sacrum is the triangular-shaped bone at the base of the spine. Stretching can help reduce any tension and pain stemming from this area of the body. Finally, I asked her if she had diarrhea. "How did you know?" she replied. Well, you can't have all the problems Melissa was having without your body and gut reacting to it.

The kind of testing I performed on Melissa was not at all what she was expecting from an orthopaedic appointment. We scheduled her for a sleep study to determine the extent of her sleep breathing issues, and she was referred to an ENT specialist to improve her breathing. We also scheduled her for a therapy program to help strengthen her core. Instead of scheduling surgery to fix her carpal tunnel symptoms, she left Romano Orthopaedic Center with most of her symptoms alleviated—including some she didn't even know about—along with instructions and a plan for how to take care of them if they returned.

Stretches to Reverse the Cubital Tunnel Reflex:

To reduce the elbow subluxation, flex the elbow to 90 degrees, then let it fall forcefully toward the ground into full extension (arm straight) with the palm facing upward. This may hurt a bit, but your pain, numbness, and tingling should decrease, and your strength should return.

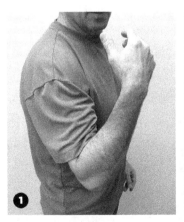 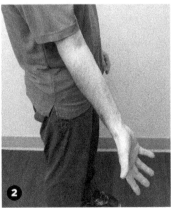

To avoid recurrent subluxation of your elbow, avoid forcefully flexing your elbow past 90 degrees, especially while exercising.

TEMPOROMANDIBULAR DISORDER (TMD)

The temporomandibular joint (TMJ) is the jaw joint located on each side of your face, just in front of your ear. When the TMJ is irritated, it is called TMD. There are many reasons for TMD, including obstructed nasal breathing, sleep apnea, bruxism (grinding your teeth while sleeping), and trauma. Most of the time, my patients are unaware they have TMD, and even remain skeptical after I point it out. Although the mind can actually shut out the joint pain, the trigeminal nerve, which lies just above the TMJ, still feels the pain. That can cause your body to go into dystrophy, making you lose your strength and balance in the dark.

I find many of my patients who visit with multiple knee injuries from noncontact sports or falls tend to have TMD. As I mentioned in chapter one, women are five to eight times more likely than men to have TMD, five to eight times more likely to have noncontact ACL tears, and they have more balance problems than men. That's more than a coincidence in my mind. That's why I believe diagnosing and treating TMD in women will improve their balance and reduce their ACL tear rate.

Some of my patients who show up with shoulder pain also have TMD. These patients tend to complain their pain is worse at night and wakes them up from sleep. Because sleep apnea is associated with TMD, sleep therapy may improve their shoulder pain symptoms.

Treating TMD is difficult. Trauma and arthritis are often responsible for TMD, as is obstructed nasal breathing, and solutions such as wearing a mouth guard to protect the teeth from grinding while sleeping only treat the symptoms. Instead, it's important to get to the underlying cause. I recommend my patients see a dentist who specializes in sleep and TMD for evaluation and treatment, perhaps get a sleep study for sleep apnea, and/or see an ENT specialist for nasal obstruction.

For athletes with TMD, having a properly fitted mouth guard is crucial for restoring balance and avoiding injury—and not just to protect the mouth and teeth. One season, I helped a soccer player after he sprained his ankle in practice. Through AMNRT testing, I determined his balance was off. I was surprised because when I had tested him before practice, his balance was perfect. I then used scratch testing and found he was positive for TMD. What changed? With the second test, he was still wearing his mouth guard; the first time I tested him, he hadn't inserted it yet. I had him remove his mouth guard, retested him, and now his balance was perfect again. Now we make sure players' mouth guards are fitted properly.

The case of another player, Shawn, who was trying to make the minor leagues in baseball, demonstrates how a properly fitted mouth guard can improve performance. He was a rising star his first two years in college and number one in hitting on his team. Unfortunately, he was plagued by multiple injuries his junior year and sat on the bench most of his senior year. He came to me for an evaluation. With AMNRT testing, I found Shawn had Morton's neuroma, CTS, obstructed breathing, and back problems. No wonder he was always injuring himself! I showed him how to fix his multiple injuries, and he was just about ready to leave my office when he mentioned he had to chew a large wad of gum to help him relax while batting. I had already tested his TMD reflex, and it was negative. On a hunch, I asked him to clench his teeth while I retested his TMD reflex. Amazingly, that made him test positive. And if he wore a mouth guard and clenched his teeth, the TMD reflex did not appear. The gum was preventing his teeth from fully clenching, thus, keeping him out of dystrophy. I'm still amazed quite often by unexpected results from AMNRT testing. In his next game, Shawn batted five for five while wearing his new performance mouth guard—and without having to chew gum.

I often refer patients with TMD to my nephew and other dentists who specialize in TMD and sleep apnea. I had the pleasure of helping my nephew fit Notre Dame athletes for these specialized protective mouth guards that enhance balance and increase strength. We actually taught a course together to the Notre Dame Sports Medicine Team illustrating AMNRT as well.

POSTERIOR RIB SUBLUXATION

Occasionally, a person's ribs can subluxate (come out of alignment), causing pain and dysfunction of the upper back. Associated symptoms include vague pain in the neck, shoulder, and/or hand; headaches; and syndromes such as rotator cuff tendinitis and tennis elbow. Rib subluxation is most common in hockey players who get checked into the boards, football players who are tackled and land on their shoulders, and heavyweight lifters. Treatment includes manipulation of the ribs, stretching the shoulders backwards in a doorway or corner of a room, proper ergonomics at work and in sports, physical therapy, and avoidance of forceful movement of the arms across the chest.

One of my patients, Andre, was a sixteen-year-old concert violinist for the youth symphony orchestra. He enjoyed practicing all day long. Unfortunately, his severe upper and lower back pain limited his ability to practice more than a half hour at a time. He also had difficulty sleeping at night. With testing, I found his upper back pain was related to subluxation (partial dislocation) of the posterior ribs, or the ribs in his back. I had him lie on his stomach, so I could manipulate his ribs on either side of his spine, which alleviated the pain in his upper back. The same result can be achieved by pulling your shoulders backwards very quickly, which is how I treat patients today.

Testing also found that the violinist's lower back pain was related to severe nasal congestion and chronically inflamed tonsils (discussed more in the next chapter). After I stretched his lower back and gave him a nasal strip, all of his pain went away. Prior to seeing me, an ENT physician had recommended nasal surgery, but they were still deciding. I encouraged him to have the surgery to alleviate his back pain. In a subsequent visit to his ENT physician, Andre's dad asked whether the nasal surgery truly would relieve his back pain, the specialist replied, "I don't know, but he'll breathe a whole lot better." Andre had the surgery. Not only did his lower back pain completely go away, but he also slept much better.

Still, before long, Andre returned to see me with persistent upper back pain. I had shown his father how to manipulate his ribs whenever Andre had pain in his upper back, but ultimately, the treatment stopped working. So, I asked Andre to simulate playing the violin loud and hard, which revealed that he swung his right arm furiously back and forth across his chest. AMNRT testing then indicated that his rib subluxation had returned. I reduced his ribs (put them back in place) and had him repeat the air-violin simulation, this time keeping his chest up and shoulders back. His smile said it all—his back pain did not return. Good posture is important.

Stretches to Reverse the Rib Subluxation Reflex:

To self-manipulate your ribs back into place, bring your elbows out to your side—parallel to the ground, and just below shoulder level—and forcefully and quickly pull your elbows backwards. You may feel some pain and discomfort, and hear an audible "pop," but you then should experience a significant reduction in symptoms.

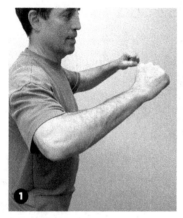 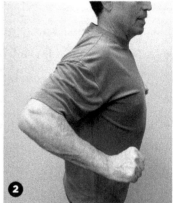

Avoid forcefully bringing your arms across your chest.

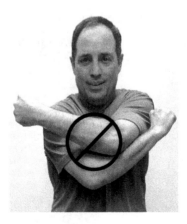

SPORTS HERNIA

A sports hernia, also called athletic pubalgia, is pain in the groin area occurring after sudden change of direction or intense twisting movement. It is commonly seen in athletes in vigorous sports, such as ice hockey, soccer, wrestling, and football. It is said to be from a strain or tear of the soft tissue in the lower abdomen or groin area.[9] However, there often is no actual tear or hernia. In fact, the diagnosis is made when there is no other cause for groin pain. If you have persistent groin pain with a negative MRI, you have a sports hernia.

I always had a hard time believing this was an accurate diagnosis. It isn't. I recently realized a sports hernia could actually be a subluxation of the symphysis pubis (the front of the pelvis).

Early last fall, I encountered a high school soccer player who had persistent groin pain for months despite rest, physical therapy, and anti-inflammatories. Testing found he was off-balance with his eyes closed, yet I could not find a positive reflex. When questioning him, he said his injury occurred when he did butterfly groin stretches after an extensive workout. So, I manipulated his pelvis by reversing the butterfly stretch, at which point I heard—and he felt—a "pop." Immediately, his pain improved significantly. He returned to his varsity soccer career. I went home and performed multiple tests on my son, Joe, who is in medical school. We used the electrical current from my cell phone to interrupt the nerve in the symphysis pubis (front of the pelvis) and discovered a new AMNRT reflex, that represents a so called "sport's hernia." Since then, I've seen and successfully treated a dozen or so people with "sports hernia" with this groin manipulation.

---

9   Justin Neal Hopkins, William Brown, and Cassandra Alda Lee, "Sports Hernia: Definition, Evaluation, and Treatment," *Journal of Bone and Joint Surgery* 5, no. 9 (September 2017), https://doi.org/10.2106/JBJS.RVW.17.00022

Stretches to Reverse the Sports Hernia Reflex:

The groin manipulation you can do yourself is actually a yoga stretch. While lying flat on your back, simply grab your knee on the affected side with your opposite arm and bring your knee toward your chest and across your body. Stretch your other arm and shoulder in the opposite direction.

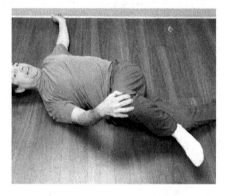

Avoid butterfly stretches. They will cause the sport's hernia reflex to reoccur.

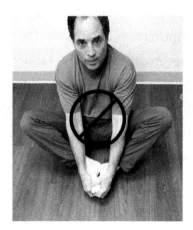

A piriformis stretch will stretch the groin and relieve pain without setting off this reflex.

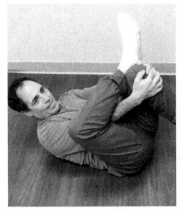 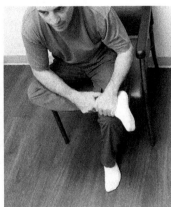

CHAPTER 3

BACK PAIN, BALANCE, BREATHING, AND STRENGTH— A STRONG CONNECTION

John is a fifty-eight-year-old firefighter, active in sports outside of work and constantly injuring himself. Over the years, I have seen John for pain in his shoulders, elbows, wrists, back, and knees. I first met him when he was in his late thirties, after he had torn his ACL playing rugby. I performed surgery on his knee, and afterward, his wife asked me in the family waiting room, "Can you tell him that he can't play rugby anymore?"

I answered, "You're too late. I already told him he will be back playing full contact in three months."

Not long after John's return to rugby, he tore his meniscus in the same knee as his new ACL. This time both his wife and his mother demanded, "You tell him no more rugby!"

What could I do? I wrote on a prescription pad, "NO MORE RUGBY!"

That note was taped on John's refrigerator door for a long time. Then one day, John told his wife he was going to work a double shift. Instead, he went out and played rugby after the first shift. Sure enough, he tore his ACL on the other knee. I heard about the injury right away but was afraid to call John at home because I knew he was trying to hide it from his wife. Of course, he couldn't. John soon came to see me with his wife. She was pretty upset but conceded, "If he wants to kill himself, let him." I fixed his ACL, and he returned to firefighting and sports soon afterwards.

He eventually had to give up rugby because of arthritis in his knees but is still competing in international strength competitions for firefighters.

Once I learned about the balance and reflex techniques I use today, I tested John and found several reflexes that were easily corrected. However, he had persistent back discomfort and weakness in his right leg. John had broken his nose so many times he only had about a 5 percent capacity to breathe through his nasal passages. That may seem unrelated, but I knew having his nasal airways open would allow his leg to get stronger. I told him so, but he insisted his breathing was fine. I even demonstrated what I meant by applying a breathing strip to his nose, which immediately opened his nasal passage. I then retested him and found that his leg was stronger.

Still, he didn't believe that his nose had anything to do with his leg weakness, so he put off nasal surgery for some time. His daughter, a physical therapist, even tried to help him regain his strength in his leg, but he never improved. Finally, he decided to undergo the surgery. After he healed, he stopped by my office and told me, "I feel like I'm breathing through a fire hose now. I wish I had listened to you before." To his surprise, his back pain also disappeared, and his balance and strength returned. That's the power of breathing.

BACK PAIN, BALANCE, BREATHING, AND STRENGTH—THE CONNECTION

Ancient Chinese medicine understood the importance of balance and breathing. However, current medical literature doesn't discuss a connection between clear nasal breathing and back pain, balance, or strength. Yet, I see it every day. Dr. Olmos has published in medical literature how he can improve a person's posture by opening the airway with jaw orthotics.[10] When I started testing my patients' balance, I found their balance and strength improved after applying nasal strips to open their airway. It's an amazing connection.

As I discussed in the last chapter, I check patients' balance first with their eyes open and then closed, to test the integrity of their peripheral nervous system. After, I check their balance with their heads turned side to side and up and down. That tests the integrity of the central nervous system.

When patients lose their balance while turning their heads, there is a problem with either the neck, upper or lower back, or sacroiliac (SI) joint, which is near the base of your spine. They have a hard time believing me, so I prove it in three ways. First, I pinpoint the exact location of the injury by pressing on certain areas along the spine while they hold their arms out against resistance. When I hit the exact source of their problem, they instantly lose their strength. They think it's a magic trick.

Secondly, I test the strength of their arms and legs in certain positions. Weakness in one position and not in another corresponds to a problem in their neck, upper or lower back, or SI joint. Now, they're really confused. Usually, they didn't realize that they had any weakness.

---

10 Steven R. Olmos et al., "The Effect of Condyle Fossa Relationships on Head Posture," *The Journal of Craniomandibular Practice* 23, no. 1 (January 2005): 48–52, https://doi.org/10.1179/crn.2005.008

Finally, I gently manipulate the source or show them how to do it themselves. Surprisingly (but not to me), their balance and strength improve, and they no longer respond to pressing along the spine.

To see if their problems are related to their breathing, I ask them to take a deep breath through the mouth. If they don't have obstructed nasal breathing, nothing happens. That means the source was along the spine, so I give them physical therapy with stretching and strengthening exercises to correct their problems and ensure their problems do not return. If they do have obstructed nasal breathing, everything returns—the loss of balance, the weakness, and the sensitivity to pressing along the spine. That usually leaves them dumbfounded, asking, "How can that be? I just breathed through my mouth!" After I give the patient a nasal breathing strip, their balance and strength return to normal and, once again, they don't respond to pressing on their spine. This is because the nasal strip mechanically opens the nasal passages and allows you to breathe easier. The weakness or loss of balance associated with nasal obstruction will subside with the nasal strip, but will return if you remove the nasal strip and start breathing through your mouth.

To help patients understand the connection between breathing and the back, I demonstrate the relationship multiple times. For instance, their balance and strength can be thrown off by blocking their nasal passage on just one side. Unblock it, and everything returns to normal. That helps them begin to understand.

Patients often ask how the connection works. The answer isn't entirely clear, but it appears to start in the womb. When a human is still just an embryo, the sympathetic chain—which controls heart rate and breathing during what is known as the "fight-or-flight" response—separates from the spinal cord five weeks after fertilization of the egg. Despite this separation, the association between clear nasal breathing and the spinal cord remains. So, if you have an obstruction of your airway and are not breathing clearly, as a result of this association, the nerves in your neck and back stop functioning at full capacity—resulting in weakness in your arms and legs. I see it every time.

A deviated septum, enlarged tonsils, or excessive inflammation in the sinuses from diet, flu, allergies, or infection can cause one or both nasal passages to completely obstruct breathing. That can lead to problems such as sleep apnea; loss of balance; pain and stiffness of the neck, upper and lower back, and pelvis; worsening back and shoulder pain at night; and weakness of the shoulders, arms, and hips.

Danny is a perfect example of the connection between nasal blockage and balance. He was an accomplished collegiate quarterback who was trying to make the last cut for a pro football team. He came to see me for lower back pain on his right side. When I asked about his balance, he was surprised because no doctor had ever tried to make that connection. He said he occasionally lost his balance when he dropped back to throw a pass, but he thought he just needed to work on his footwork. Instead, I found when he turned his neck to the left, he lost his balance due to a back and balance reflex associated with his lower back pain on the right side. I also found that he had right shoulder weakness, which he didn't report. The solutions to his problems were proper stretching and a simple nasal strip. It helped him so much he swore he would never play without a nasal strip again. Unfortunately, he didn't make the last cut for his pro team, but fortunately for us, he is now pursuing a career in medicine instead.

TROUBLE BREATHING AT NIGHT? MIGHT BE SLEEP APNEA

Patients with blocked nasal passages have a high likelihood of having obstructive sleep apnea (OSA). OSA occurs when the soft tissue in the back of the throat narrows and repeatedly closes during sleep, causing that all-too-familiar snoring you may have heard in others. With OSA, breathing can stop for anywhere from ten to sixty seconds. These apnea events (breaks in breathing) may occur five to fifty times per hour. The brain responds to each of these events by waking the apnea sufferer to resume breathing. Because apnea events can happen hundreds of times per night, sleep becomes broken and ineffective, and this can lead to serious health consequences. There are several reasons why, as an orthopaedist, I am so concerned about sleep apnea.

First, sleep apnea is prevalent everywhere. It is estimated that up to 26 percent of adults may have sleep apnea, 80 to 90 percent which is unrecognized.[11] Two NFL studies demonstrated a 14 percent incidence of sleep apnea in current players, with a 34 percent incidence in linemen and a 52 percent incidence in retired NFL players.[12] Untreated sleep apnea can lead to poor performance on and off the playing field, as well as more injuries.[13] Compared to

---

11   Paul E. Peppard, "Increased prevalence of sleep-disordered breathing in adults," *American Journal of Epidemiology* 77, no. 9 (May 1, 2013):1006–14, https://doi.org/10.1093/aje/kws342

12   Charles F.P. George et al., "Increased Prevalence of Sleep-Disordered Breathing among Professional Football Players," *New England Journal of Medicine* 56, no. 17 (January 23, 2003): 367–368, https://doi.org/10.1056/NEJM200301233480422; Felipe N. Albuquerque et al., "Sleep-Disordered Breathing, Hypertension, and Obesity in RetiredNational Football League Players," *Journal of the American College of Cardiology* 56, no. 17 (October 2010): 1432–1433, https://doi.org/10.1016/j.jacc.2010.03.099

13   N.S. Simpson, E.L. Gibbs, and Gordon Matheson, "Optimizing sleep to maximize performance: implications and recommendations for elite

people without sleep apnea, workers with sleep apnea are two times more likely to suffer an injury at work.[14] Truck drivers with sleep apnea are seven times more likely to get into a preventable crash.[15]

Second, sleep apnea leads to high blood pressure, depression, diabetes, heart disease, atrial fibrillation (abnormal heart rhythm), stroke, erectile dysfunction, and early dementia.[16] If I can help my patients avoid any of these problems, why wouldn't I?

Third, the body needs at least seven hours of sleep per day to be fully refreshed.[17] If you aren't sleeping well, how is your back or shoulder injury going to get better? Studies show that not breathing for an extended period will severely exacerbate your pain.[18] And both pain medication and sleeping pills can worsen your sleep apnea,

athletes," *Scandinavian Journal of Medicine & Science in Sports* 27, no. 3 (March 2017): 266–274, https://doi.org/10.1111/sms.12703

14   Sergio Garbarino et al., "Risk of Occupational Accidents in Workers With Obstructive Sleep Apnea: Systematic Review and Meta-analysis," *Sleep* 39, no. 6 (June 1, 2016): 1211-8, https://doi.org/10.5665/sleep.5834

15   Guang X. Chen, Harlan Amandus, and Nan Wu, "Occupational Fatalities Among Driver/Sales Workers and Truck Drivers in the United States, 2003 – 2008," *American Journal of Industrial Medicine* 57, no. 7 (July 2014): 800–9, https://doi.org/10.1002/ajim.22320

16   "Sleep Apnea," Mayo Clinic, https://www.mayoclinic.org/diseases-con-ditions/sleep-apnea/symptoms-causes/syc-20377631; Daniel J. Gottlieb, "Sleep Apnea and the Risk of Atrial Fibrillation Recurrence: Structural of Functional Effects?" *Journal of the American Heart Association* 3, no. 1 (January 2014), https://doi.org/10.1161/JAHA.113.000654; Farnoosh Emamian et al., "The Association Between Obstructive Sleep Apnea and Alzheimer's Disease: A Meta-Analysis Perspective," *Frontiers in Aging Neuroscience* 8 (April 12, 2016), https://doi.org/10.3389/fnagi.2016.00078; Kerem Taken et al., "Erectile dysfunction is a marker for obstructive sleep apnea," *The Aging Male* 19, no. 2 (June 2016): 102–105, https://doi.org/10.31 09/13685538.2015.1131259

17   "National Sleep Foundation Recommends New Sleep Times," National Sleep Foundation, https://sleepfoundation.org/press-release/national-sleep-foundation-recommends-new-sleep-times/page/0/1

18   Christopher J. Lettieri, "The Association of Obstructive Sleep Apnea and Chronic Pain," *Medscape*, May 24, 2013, https://www.medscape.com/viewarticle/804588

increasing your risk of complications without significantly improving your pain.

Finally, orthopaedic patients with sleep apnea are at a higher risk for postoperative complications (up to 43 percent) than patients who do not have sleep apnea.[19] They are more likely to experience respiratory and cardiac complications (pneumonia, pulmonary embolism, cardiac arrest, stroke, shock, or sudden death), be transferred to an intensive care unit, or have a longer hospital stay. Administration of anesthesia, sedatives, narcotics, and muscle relaxants increases the risk of these complications. These risks markedly diminish when patients are actively treated for sleep apnea.

Symptoms of sleep apnea include excessive daytime sleepiness, heavy snoring, frequent awakening at night, using the restroom at night, poor concentration, morning headaches, moodiness, and irritability. Children with sleep apnea may have snoring, learning disabilities, attention deficit hyperactivity disorder (ADHD), bedwetting, teeth grinding, and night terrors. There are a number of risk factors that can cause or contribute to sleep apnea, including obesity, hypertension, alcohol use, smoking, family history of sleep apnea, large neck size, nasal obstruction, and chronic respiratory problems. Sleep apnea is confirmed via a diagnostic sleep study, either at home or in a sleep center. Treatment consists of using a CPAP machine during sleep or wearing an oral appliance to prevent collapse of the airway while sleeping. Sometimes, corrective nasal surgery is necessary.

---

19   Syed Yaseeen Naqvi et al., "Perioperative Complications in Patients with Sleep Apnea Undergoing Total Joint Arthoplasty," *The Journal of Arthoplasty* 32, no.9 (September 2017): 2680–2683, https://doi.org/10.1016/j.arth.2017.04.040

NASAL BLOCKAGE AND BACK PAIN—THREE CASE STUDIES

As further proof of the connection between nasal blockage and back pain, let me tell you about three different patients of mine.

Otto was an Austrian nurse, a big guy who resembled Arnold Schwarzenegger—but without the muscles. While working in a nursing home, Otto was assaulted by one of the residents—a seventy-year-old US Marine. Since Otto was such a large man, it seemed like he could've handled himself well enough.

However, when Otto came to see me, he complained of pain and weakness all over his body. He had already undergone three MRI studies, none of which found a source of the pain. I was his third orthopaedist. The two before me did not want to treat Otto because he had a 100 percent invalid score on a functional capacity evaluation (FCE). An FCE measures a patient's strength and gives a validity score to measure their effort. It's a useful test for workers' compensation claims to determine whether the patient can return to work that requires a specific level of strength and to see if they are giving their best effort. Until Otto, I had never seen a 100 percent invalid score—in workers' compensation claims, that kind of score can indicate someone who is faking their injury or inability.

Otto, however, had multiple positive AMNRT balance tests, and I detected obstructed breathing with associated weakness—these cannot be faked. I also identified he potentially had sleep-disorder breathing issues (which turned out to be sleep apnea). With appropriate therapy, a lot of his pain went away, but his back pain still kept him out of work. He eventually had nasal surgery (which was approved through workers' compensation, although with some difficulty), and his back pain went away. Soon afterwards, he returned to full-time work as a nurse.

As another example, Drew, a twenty-five-year-old golfer who is trying to break into the pro tour, came to see me for back pain. Along with a pelvic tilt with associated left-sided weakness and a stiff right shoulder (see chapter four), I found he lost his balance when he bent his head down and had associated weakness of his right shoulder. That's a problem for a golfer trying to address the ball. Drew told me he knew about the balance problem but not about the weakness. Because of his balance issue, he was forcefully keeping his neck straight and only moved his eyes downward to take a shot. I gave him a nasal strip, and he finally could flex his neck without losing his balance. Of course, he was excited he could look down on the ball naturally for each shot. I also recommended he see a specialist to permanently fix his chronic nasal congestion, in part because he reported having difficulty sleeping. No doubt, a good night's sleep would help his game, too.

One more example: Ava was an eleven-year-old swimmer who saw me for asymptomatic scoliosis (non-painful curvature in her spine). Her spine measured a 22 degree curve, which was noted by her pediatrician during her back-to-school physical. She reported occasional lower back pain—a one to two out of ten on a pain scale—only on waking and blamed it on her mattress. Her dad, however, noted she had difficulty waking up in the morning and ground her teeth at night. She had not been diagnosed with ADHD, but her dad reported she had behavioral problems and difficulty concentrating in school. She also had seasonal allergies for which she did not take any medication.

When I examined her, I did find the gentle curve of the spine, but it was not tender. However, AMNRT balance testing revealed she had TMD, and her breathing and back testing revealed nasal congestion on the left side, with associated left lower back tenderness. She had a pelvic tilt on the left, which improved with stretching (see chapter four). Remarkably, both her TMD and lower back pathologic reflexes cleared with a nasal strip. She was so excited with her wide-open breathing she wouldn't take the nasal strip off. She just smiled and kept on saying, "Wow!"

Normally, with a 22 degree curve, I would have done nothing but have her return in three or four months for a repeat X-ray. If her curvature ever progressed to 30 degrees or more, she would be required to wear a back brace for about two years until she stops growing. Instead, I gave her a stretching program for her lower back and instructions on clearing her sinuses using allergy medication and saline rinses. I also asked her parents to monitor her sleep. If she fails to improve, I will send her for a sleep study and a referral to an ENT and/or dental sleep specialist. Hopefully, her spinal curve will improve along with her attention in school and overall health.

Methods to Improve Breathing and Performance:

Clearing the nasal passage and keeping it clear will reverse the balance loss with head turning, relieve neck and back symptoms and restore strength in the arms and legs. Methods I recommend include the following:

- **Nasal strips**: You may have seen these advertised for snoring relief and worn by football players on the field. These strips can be worn at nighttime and during exercise. They work by opening your nasal passage, allowing you to breathe and sleep better. They even may help relieve your lower back and upper arm pain. Note: If the strips won't stay on your nose, or if the tape irritates your skin, try nasal cones or nasal dilators instead.

- **Nasal rinse and Neti pot**: These involve pouring a saline solution into one nostril with your head tilted, and then letting the liquid run out of your opposite nostril. This method is best used at bedtime and/or after you wake up.

- **Nasal sprays**: Steroid, antihistamine, and saline sprays can all open your nasal passage. Some can be used several times throughout the day, as needed.

- **Cold and allergy medicine:** Be sure it includes a decongestant if you need it.

If these methods do not improve your breathing and sleep and reverse the problem reflexes, you may need to see an ENT specialist and/or a dental sleep specialist to help diagnose and correct your obstruction and relieve your pain.

Neck Stretches:

To stretch your neck, bring your neck all the way back over your shoulders, and then slowly lift your chin upward, tilting your head as far back as possible. Repeat two more times.

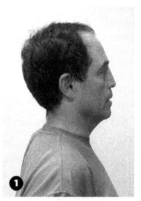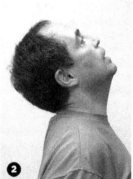

Another good neck stretch is to bring your head back and then tuck your chin down as far as possible. Next, slowly rotate your neck away from the sore side in a clockwise or counterclockwise direction while reaching as far as possible in each direction.

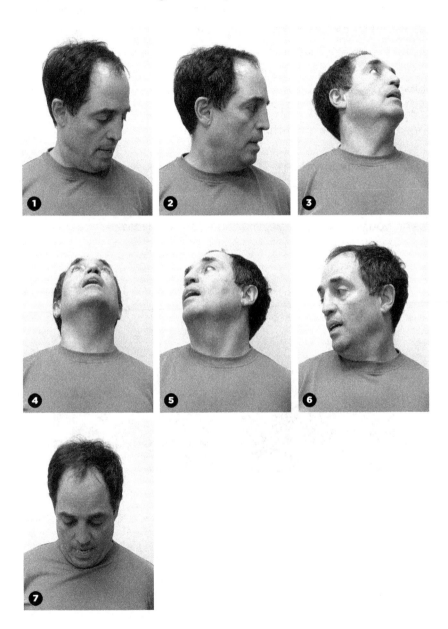

Stretching Exercises for the Neck and Back:

If your back and/or neck are out of alignment, stretching and mobilizing the SI joint, upper and lower back, and neck will reverse the loss of balance with head turning, relieve neck and back symptoms, and restore strength in the arms and legs associated with your malalignment. However, if the above problems are associated with blocked nasal passages, your neck and back symptoms, along with your loss of balance and strength, will return as soon as you breathe once through your mouth.

Lumbar Spine Stretches: To stretch your lumbar spine on the right side, bring your right leg up on a chair or step behind you and arch your back to get a good stretch in your hip flexors. Then slowly bend your left knee to get a deeper stretch. Hold for a slow count of three, and repeat two more times.

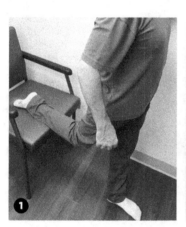 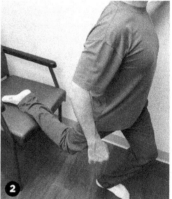

SI Joint Stretches: This is the same stretch as the sports hernia stretch described in chapter two. While lying flat on your back, simply grab your knee on the affected side with your opposite arm and bring your knee toward your chest and across your body. Stretch your other arm and shoulder in the opposite direction.

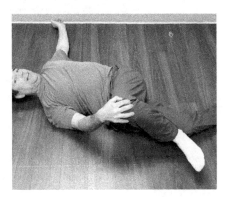

Override Stretch for Obstructive Breathing Problems:

Interestingly enough, I have found a temporary bypass for obstructed breathing and back pain—a workaround, if you will. Hyperextending (arching) your back will temporarily override these reflexes. It's a pretty simple stretch, and the results last for approximately one hour.

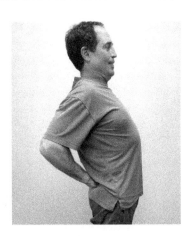

Once the loss of balance from the peripheral nerves and central nerves have been identified and treated, the next neuromuscular system to assess is the patient's core because the trunk must be stable to support the limbs.

CHAPTER 4

A LEVEL PELVIS—THE KEY TO CORE STABILITY AND BALANCE

Although I don't take credit for the successful 2016 football season of the Fenwick High School Friars of Oak Park, Illinois, I do take credit for keeping our players on the field.

Conner was our star running back. Late in the season, he was tackled early in the game and came down hard on his shoulder. I was late to the game, arriving shortly after his injury, so the school's athletic trainer had examined Conner instead. Conner had tenderness over his acromioclavicular (AC) joint (on top of the shoulder) and was diagnosed with an AC separation. The trainer wrapped Conner's shoulder in ice and shut him down for the game, then told the coach it would be weeks before he could return. An AC separation is a very painful injury. I had the same injury while playing rugby in college and was out for several games. It bothered me for the rest of the season.

During halftime, I examined Conner and found that his AC joint was tender and mildly swollen. But my balance assessment determined the source of his pain was his lower back. His SI joint was tilted. After stretching his lower back, which leveled his pelvis, most of Conner's pain went away. So, he suited up for the second half and scored two touchdowns in our first two possessions. The Friars won easily. Afterward, while reviewing the game films of his injury, I could see that, although he landed on his shoulder, his back had twisted significantly.

In a similar incident the year prior, our wide receiver, Kirk, was down on the field complaining of shoulder pain. At the time, I was tending to a cheerleader who fell during a routine, so another orthopaedist, who Kirk had seen before and also was on the sidelines, went to look him over. The orthopaedist determined Kirk had a shoulder sprain and told the coach he would be out for at least two games. I didn't want to contradict my colleague, so I didn't examine Kirk.

The next day in the training room, I determined the source of Kirk's injury was his lower back. After he stretched his lower back, his shoulder pain went away. As a result, he didn't miss one day of practice.

A few games later, however, Kirk again came off the field complaining of shoulder pain when there were only a few minutes left to go in the game. The team was down by six points, and my colleague mentioned it was probably the same shoulder injury. This time I didn't listen to him. Instead, I examined Kirk and helped him stretch his lower back. He immediately felt better and went back into the game. Two plays later, Kirk was in the end zone and reached up with his injured shoulder and grabbed the ball above the heads of the two opponents to score the winning goal—except he dropped the ball when he brought it back down. Game over. Fenwick lost. Still, thanks to stretching and balance testing, Kirk came out a winner— he didn't miss a game all season.

YOU NEED A STRONG CORE

After I test the peripheral nervous system (see chapter two) and the central nervous system (chapter three), the final area I test for balance is the pelvis.

The core of the body is the center of strength. All functional movement begins at the core. Weakness of the core predisposes a person to injuries in other areas of the body. The core muscles align the spine, ribs, and pelvis, stabilizing the body.

Normally, the pelvis is level and parallel to the ground. When it's level, the body is in alignment; you feel good and everything works. Occasionally, with tightness or spasms in the lower back, the pelvis can be tilted or "out of alignment." This causes one leg to appear longer than the other, a fairly common condition that is normally not a major problem. In fact, it's rare one leg is physically longer than the other; usually the problem is a tilted pelvis.

About one-third of my patients have this condition, but their bodies compensate for it. They're always protecting what is actually a weak core. People with a pelvic tilt often go on about their day normally. However, pelvic tilt leads to side-to-side instability. When I test patients with pelvic tilt, I find they're unstable and their side-to-side balance is off—that's how I can push a 300-pound man off-balance. So, when something out of the ordinary happens—even a misstep or a slight turn the wrong way—people with this condition tend to injure themselves.

Pelvic tilt with subsequent leg length discrepancy can also lead to lower back pain. In one study of more than four hundred patients with back pain, 80 percent had a leg length discrepancy of greater than or equal to 4 millimeters, 50 percent had a 10-millimeter discrepancy, and 20 percent had a 15-millimeter discrepancy.[20]

Another disorder associated with pelvic tilt I see occasionally is piriformis syndrome, which occurs when the piriformis muscle,

---

20 John Henry Juhl, Tonya M. Ippolito Cremin, and George Russell, "Prevalence of Frontal Plane Pelvic Postural Asymmetry—Part 1," *The Journal of the American Osteopathic Association* 104, no. 10 (October 2004): 411–421, http://jaoa.org/article.aspx?articleid=2092944

a small muscle in the buttocks, causes pain and even may irritate the sciatic nerve. With piriformis syndrome, the body often over compensates for the weak pelvic tilt side and ultimately abuses the piriformis on the opposite side.

Sciatica is another condition I sometimes see in patients with a pelvic tilt. Sciatica is characterized by pain shooting down the leg from the lower back. The pain travels down the sciatic nerve, hence the name.

Diagnosing pelvic tilt can be as easy as looking at the patient from behind. With severe pelvic tilt, the evidence is clear. However, sometimes a patient's pelvis appears level but when they bend over and I place my thumbs on their pelvis, I can see one side moving more than the other. When I'm testing for side-to-side balance, I stand next to the patient, who is standing upright (not leaning), and tug on the patient's arm. If the pelvis is tilted, he or she will not be able to remain upright on the side of the pelvis that is higher, but will remain rigid when I tug on the lower side. With elderly patients, I just lean on them a little—they can hold me up when I lean on the low side but can't on the high side. The good news is that with a few adjustments, they can leave the office feeling great and with better balance.

With pelvic tilt, if one has pain, the pain is usually at the SI joint. SI joint pain is in the lower back and buttocks and can extend down the leg. The pain can worsen with prolonged sitting, standing, or climbing stairs. Common causes are trauma, arthritis, obesity, pregnancy, and repetitive stress from activities like running or jumping.

The major muscles involved in the core are the pelvic floor muscles, abdominal muscles, paraspinal muscles (on either side of the spine), and the largest muscle of the core, the diaphragm (which controls your breathing). When strengthening the core, the diaphragm is often overlooked. As discussed in chapter three, breathing is important in stabilizing the spine. As the Chinese understood thousands of years ago, diaphragmatic breathing is important and will reverse weaknesses when the spine is out of alignment.

Although the latissimus dorsi is considered a minor core muscle, it is the link from the core to the shoulder. *Latissimus* means "broadest." As its name implies, it is the broadest muscle of the back, originating from the spine and attaching to the upper arm. A powerful muscle, it brings the shoulder close to the body. Asymmetrical weakness of the latissimus dorsi, when holding the arm tight toward the side, suggests the pelvis is out of alignment. With latissimus dorsi weakness, lateral core stability on the affected side is significantly diminished, and shoulder motion is restricted, increasing the risk of injury.

Pelvic tilt is often overlooked. Since my first experience with AMNRT, I routinely witness the association of dysfunction of the pelvis with weakness, neck pain, and pain and stiffness of the opposite shoulder.

Reduced range of motion in the shoulder is common in overhead athletes. The problem in baseball is that pitchers who do not have full shoulder range of motion miss more games from injuries than pitchers who have full range of motion.[21] With the help of my son, I recently performed a double-blind study with a minor-league baseball team (to be presented to the American Academy of Ortho-paedic Surgeons in New Orleans). We initially measured the players' internal shoulder range of motion (how far they could rotate their shoulders toward their bodies while supine) in their throwing arm, compared to the range of motion in their non-dominant arm. Not

---

21   L.U. Bigliani et at., "Shoulder motion and laxity in the professional baseball player," *The American Journal of Sports Medicine* 25, no. 5 (September–October 1997): 609–13, https://doi.org/10.1177/036354659702500504

surprisingly, we found most players had less internal rotation on their throwing arm. For the study, half of them stretched their throwing arm using the "gold standard" sleeper's stretch, which is performed by lying on their side and using one hand to push their opposite arm toward the ground. The other half of the athletes stretched their SI joints opposite their dominant shoulders. Internal range of motion improved twice as much in the group that stretched the opposite SI joint when compared to the group that stretched their shoulder. This had never been demonstrated before.

After this study, I learned a 2013 study reported that professional baseball players with shoulder injuries and decreased external rotation of their shoulders also had hip flexion contractures on the same side. So, I began testing my own patients and found that to be true. Then, I went one step further. I had my patients with loss of shoulder external rotation stretch their hip flexors on the same side. Remarkably, most of them had improvement of external rotation of their shoulder afterwards.

While assessing patients with shoulder pain, I always check the range of motion of their shoulder and their lower back. If they have a loss of shoulder internal rotation, I usually see tilting of the pelvis on the opposite side. In addition, if they have a loss of shoulder external rotation, I usually see tightness of their hip flexors on the same side. Furthermore, if I reverse the pelvic tilt by stretching the SI joint and if I stretch their hip flexors, their shoulder rotation improves dramatically. My patients find it incredible, because it works!

To get lasting results, an aggressive stretching and strengthening program and physical therapy is often necessary. Occasionally, I have to inject the SI joint, but only as a last resort.

Stretching and Strengthening for Pelvic Tilt:

It is essential to stretch and stabilize the core. Here are some exercises you can do on your own.

Yoga stretches: Lie flat on your back. Grab your knee on the affected side and pull it toward the opposite shoulder. Hold for a slow count of ten. Then reposition your leg flat, and relax. Repeat this stretch two more times. After the third set, keep holding your knee with the opposite arm from the knee and bring it across your body. Release your other arm from your knee and bring it out to your side. Hold for a slow count of ten. Switch sides. Do this before you get out of bed in the morning, when you go to bed at night, and several times during the day.

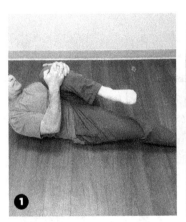 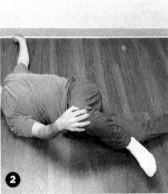

Rotational stretches: Hip rotations and toe touches also will help level your spine and restore balance. Rotate your hips side to side twenty times while periodically bending down to touch your toes.

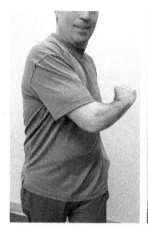 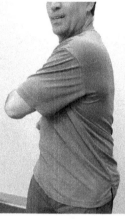 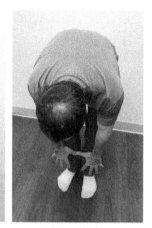

For hip flexion tightness: To stretch your hip flexors on the right side, bring your right leg up on a chair or step behind you and arch your back to get a good stretch in your hip flexors. Then slowly bend your left knee to get a deeper stretch. Hold for a slow count of three and repeat two more times. Reverse the stretch with your left leg on a chair and slowly bend your right knee for three sets.

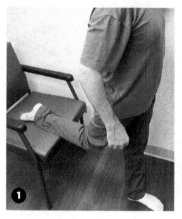 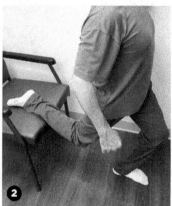

For Strengthening of the Core:

Back bridges: Start by lying flat on the floor or bed with your arms to your sides, then bend your knees to position your feet under your knees and raise your back and bottom off the floor as high as you can. Repeat several times.

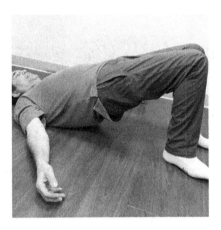

Wall lifts: Standing against a wall, lift your leg closest to the wall 90 degrees. Place a pillow between your knee and the wall, and push your knee against the wall. Hold for as long as you can. This stabilizes the pelvis on the opposite side.

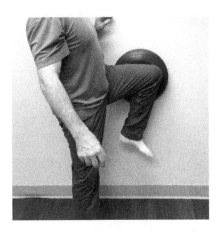

Pelvic planks: Planks are another core-stabilizing exercise that can help prevent pelvic tilt from returning. Simply prop yourself up on your toes, support your upper body placing your elbows underneath your shoulders, and keep your body as straight as possible.

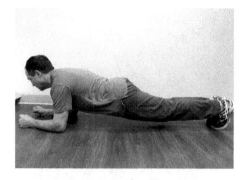

Now, let's look at ways to keep your joints healthy, what you can do to avoid joint replacements, and how to know when you really do need replacements.

CHAPTER 5
BETTER JOINTS, FEWER REPLACEMENT SURGERIES

Curtis was fifty years old when I replaced both of his degenerating knees. He had just retired from the post office after thirty years of delivering mail door-to-door. Work was getting too hard for him because of his painful knees, so he decided to take early retirement, fix his knees, and move on to the next chapter of his life.

Curtis first came to see me ten years earlier, requesting bilateral knee replacements. He was of average height and a little overweight, with bowed legs and minimally swollen knees. Although he had been bowlegged all his life, his bowing was getting worse. He had full range of motion in both knees and normal strength. While in high school, Curtis had undergone surgery on both of his knees. He did well afterwards but had been having intermittent discomfort in both knees for the previous two years. He came to see me because his primary care physician told him he needed bilateral knee replacements. X-rays showed a near-complete collapse of the cartilage on the inside half of both knees with moderate degenerative changes.

At that time, I told Curtis he was too young for knee replacements and we would proceed with aggressive yet conservative care for as long as possible. He would improve, I told him, under my care. Eventually he would need knee replacements, but not at that first visit. However, I also told him whenever he had enough, he could simply tell me it was time to replace both knee joints, and I would do the surgery as soon as possible, no questions asked. A little disappointed at first, he decided to trust me and proceed with my recommendations.

On that first visit, I gave him bilateral knee injections, started him on an aggressive course of physical therapy, changed his arthritis medication, and recommended over-the-counter supplements. He also began a home exercise program and changed his diet, which included cutting out the regular soda pop and processed foods, and instead drinking low-fat milk, taking vitamin D, and eating more nutritious foods including fruits and vegetables. Losing several pounds and keeping it off, he did very well and continued delivering the mail "through rain or shine." For ten years, he came to see me regularly for steroid injections and injections of lubricating gel into both knees. At some point, I gave him bilateral knee braces that unloaded the collapsed medial side of his knees and put his weight on the good cartilage on the outside of the knees. He wore the braces periodically during the early days of his treatment, but toward the end of his career, he had started to wear them all day at work.

Right before his fiftieth birthday, Curtis told me, "It's time." If I had replaced both of his knees on his first visit like he had wanted me to do, he probably would have been coming to me for bilateral revision surgery for his fiftieth birthday instead. Revision surgery is a lot more difficult. The prostheses must be removed and replaced, and chances are some of his bone would have also been worn down and need replacing too. That would have been a much more difficult surgery, and the results would not have been as good.

I replaced both of his knees at the same time. He recovered very well. After two days, he was out of the hospital and walking with a cane. Benefitting from ten years of improved technology, he received the next generation of total knee implants, which most likely will be his last. He is now set to enjoy a pain-free and active retirement.

TOTAL JOINT REPLACEMENTS—PROS AND CONS

The joint is the connection between two bones, allowing the body to move and function. The joint cartilage (articular cartilage) is a self-lubricating, thick layer of tissue that covers and protects the ends of the bones of the joint. Cartilage allows the shoulder, elbow, hip, knee, and ankle joints to bear heavy loads while moving precisely, almost without friction.

Damage to the articular cartilage, muscles, or bones surrounding the joint can lead to arthritis, which is the leading cause of disability in people over age fifty-five. The most common form is osteoarthritis. Otherwise known as degenerative joint disease, osteoarthritis is the loss of cartilage from infection, trauma, or simply the wear and tear of a long and active life. Because cartilage does not have a blood or nerve supply, damage to it may not be felt for hours or even until the next day after an injury. Unlike other tissues in the body, articular cartilage is limited in how it can repair itself. Arthritis is not something that can be removed with surgery or scraped out with a scope, so it is best to preserve the cartilage as long as possible. That means you must listen to your joints. Don't keep running when your knees are telling you to stop!

My approach to total joint replacements is very conservative. Although I am a surgeon, I believe surgery only should be done when necessary and as a last resort. Total joint replacements are wonderful and can be life changing. However, on rare occasions, they also can be painful, wear down prematurely, and become infected. We take great precautions to prevent infection, including daily scrubs with antibiotic soap before surgery, appropriate and timely antibiotics, recommending good dental care before surgery (to prevent an infected tooth from infecting the new joint), meticulous operative techniques and sterility precautions, silver-coated dressings, and short hospital stays.

Unfortunately, prostheses wear down. A total joint replacement in a seventy-year-old patient will last approximately fifteen years. With the average life expectancy being eighty-five years, chances are this would be the only knee replacement the patient would need. For a forty-year-old who is much more active than a seventy-year-old, a knee replacement may last only ten years.

"No problem, go ahead and replace the knee again in ten years," some patients say. Big problem! The total knee replacement consists of metal moving on plastic. Like the heel of your shoe, the plastic will wear down over time. The more active you are, the faster the plastic will wear down. Add obesity to the equation, and the plastic will wear down even more.

The problem is the plastic debris. As you may know, plastic in the environment doesn't break down. A thousand years from now, the world's garbage will be a huge problem because of the accumulation of plastic debris. The same happens in a knee replacement. Over time, the plastic debris accumulates in the knee joint. The more active you are, and the more you weigh, the more plastic debris. The white cells in your body recognize that plastic debris as foreign invaders and try to break it down. The more debris, the greater the number of white cells. Since the white cells can't break down the plastic, they instead will attack the surrounding bone. Therefore, when it becomes time to replace the plastic joint, we will also have to replace the bone. That is a significant surgery I don't enjoy, and I guarantee you won't either.

The best approach for arthritis of the knee is to wait as long as possible before replacing the knee. That way, the replaced joint won't have to last as long. Furthermore, the longer you wait, the more science will advance, and the better the knee replacements will be.

Still, I've had patients say, "I see on the Internet that they have new knee replacements that will last thirty years." Do you believe everything you see on the Internet? Although technology is improving daily, the knee replacements they may have heard about haven't been around for thirty years. It's better to wait a little while to make sure they prove themselves. When it comes time for a knee replacement, I will give you the best one available at that time.

EIGHT STEPS FOR DEALING WITH ARTHRITIS

My approach to arthritis is also conservative. I recommend eight steps for dealing with it before surgery. The first seven you can do on your own, without the aid of a medical professional.

1. Wear good shoes with arch supports.

With weight bearing and time, the arches in feet tend to fail. Good shoes with arch supports improve the alignment of the feet and ultimately improve the alignment of the knees. In addition, the feet and ankles act as shock absorbers for the knees. The better the shoes, the less stress on your knees. These are the arch supports I recommend:

- Spenco, Sof Sole, or Superfeet: These are the best of the soft insoles ($20–$40).

- Dr. Scholl's Custom Fit Orthotic Inserts: These are computer-fitted arch supports available through Walmart and Walgreens ($50).

2. Use a hinged knee brace, as needed, for support.

Although a knee sleeve with a hole for the kneecap may be enough to relieve some stress to your knee, a hinged knee brace may be even better. The best is a hinged knee brace that unloads the arthritic area and allows you to pursue more pain-free activities, which you may not have been able to do otherwise. The sturdier the brace, the bulkier it will be. I recommend you wear the smallest brace that makes you the most comfortable. Do not wear the brace for everyday activities but for extra activities, such as shopping, golfing, or exercise. You may as well be as comfortable as you can.

Bob, a fifty-year-old executive, came to see me looking for an alternative to a knee replacement. He had been told by a couple of orthopaedists he had no other options but surgery. I gave him an unloader knee brace, and he was thrilled. An avid hunter, he was able to return to his sport without pain and without surgery.

Note: If you need a brace as soon as you get up in the morning and take it off before you go to bed, it may be time to get a knee replacement.

3. Try over-the-counter pain medication and anti-inflammatories for pain or discomfort.

(If these do not suffice, consider speaking with your doctor about prescription medications.)

- **Tylenol (acetaminophen)**
  - 500 mg every 6 hours
  - Maximum dosage: 2,000 mg in 24 hours.
  - Beware of other medications that contain acetaminophen; too much acetaminophen may damage your liver.

- **Nonsteroidal anti-inflammatory drugs (NSAIDs)**
  - Advil (ibuprofen)

    1 tablet, 200 mg each, every 4 – 6 hours

    Maximum dosage: 1,200 mg (6 tablets) in 24 hours
  - Aleve (naproxen)

    1 tablet, 220 mg each, every 8 – 12 hours

    Maximum dosage: 660 mg (3 tablets) in 24 hours
  - Note: Do not mix NSAIDs. NSAIDs should be taken with food. Beware of possible side effects, including an upset stomach and bloody or dark, tarry stools. If you have these symptoms, stop taking the NSAID immediately and contact your physician. If you are taking NSAIDs for an extended period, consider taking Pepcid or an over-the-counter proton-pump inhibitor to protect your stomach from ulcers.
- **Topical pain-relieving creams**
  - Cortisone, Aspercreme, Arnica
  - Lidocaine (can be mixed with the above topical creams)

4. Take dietary supplements.

- **Glucosamine sulfate and Chondrointin sulfate**: Key components in cartilage, glucosamine and chondroitin sulfate aid in rebuilding and repairing worn cartilage. The effectiveness of these supplements is constantly under debate since they are sold "over the counter" in North America (and are typically not of pharmaceutical grade), whereas they are registered drugs in Europe.

  Although the Glucosamine/chondroitin Arthritis Trial (GAIT) study, the largest randomized controlled trial in North America, did not report any significant effect for glucosamine in patients with osteoarthritis of the knee when compared to celecoxib, a prescription NSAID, I still recommend them.[22] Oral NSAIDs have well known side-effects, especially in older patients and in patients with gastrointestinal, cardiac and kidney diseases. On the other hand, the side-effects of glucosamine and chondroitin are minimal. So why not take them?

European studies stress the importance of pharmaceutical grade products rather than food supplements.[23] A recent study shows pharmaceutical-grade chondroitin sulfate as effective as a celecoxib and more effective than placebo.[24]

- I recommend buying a two-month supply of glucosamine sulfate—not glucosamine HCL (read the label carefully)—and chondroitin sulfate. If it yields positive results after two months, great—continue taking them. If not, stop.

- If you are a long-distance runner or have had meniscus surgery, take glucosamine as a preventive measure. It can't hurt.

---

22 Allen D. Sawitzke et al., "Clinical efficacy and safety of glucosamine, chondroitin sulphate, their combination, celecoxib or placebo taken to treat osteoarthritis of the knee: 2-year results from GAIT," *Annals of the Rheumatic Diseases* 69, no. 8 (August 2010):1459–64, https://doi.org/10.1136/ard.2009.120469

23 Yves Henrotin, Marc Marty, Ali Mobasheri, "What is the current status of chondroitin sulfate and glucosamine for the treatment of knee osteoarthritis?" *Maturitas* 78, no. 3 (July 2014):184–7, https://doi.org/10.1016/j.maturitas.2014.04.015

24 Jean-Yves Reginster et al., "Pharmaceutical-grade Chondroitin sulfate is as effective as celecoxib and superior to placebo in symptomatic knee osteoarthritis: the ChONdroitin versus CElecoxib versus Placebo Trial (CONCEPT)," *Annals of the Rheumatic Diseases* 76, no. 9 (September 2017):1537–1543, https://www.ncbi.nlm.nih.gov/pubmed/8533290

- **Omega 3/fish oil**
  - Dosage: 2,000 mg, 2 times/day
  - Omega 3 has been shown to help your heart, brain, and joints. It's a three-for-one deal. Why not take it?
- **Vitamin D3** (See chapter six.)
  - Dosage: 2,000 – 4,000 IU/day
- **Dietary calcium** (See chapter six.)
  - Dosage: 1,200 mg/day

5. Have a daily exercise and balance program.

As they say, use it or lose it! Studies show that arthritic patients who exercise do much better than those who don't.[25] I recommend at least a twenty-minute daily exercise program for all patients with arthritis.

Remember the old saying, "No pain, no gain"? That's old school. Pain is telling you, "Stop! You're hurting your joints." Exercise should not be painful and should include stretching, aerobic activity, and strength training. If certain physical activities or exercises cause discomfort, you should try something else or consult a physical therapist or orthopaedist to see if they can help. In addition, our AMNRT and balance-testing program will help optimize your core strength and balance.

6. Eat nutritious foods, and keep your weight in check.

Have you ever been in this scenario?

Doctor: "Does carrying groceries up the stairs hurt your knees?"

Patient: "I never do that, it hurts too much."

---

25   Linda Fernandes et al., "EULAR recommendations for the non-pharmacological core management of hip and knee osteoarthritis," *Annals of the Rheumatic Diseases* (April 17, 2013) http://doi.org/10.1136/annrheumdis-2012-202745

Doctor: "Why is that?"

Patient: "Too much weight."

Doctor: "Exactly! That's why if you lose a 'few bags of groceries,' your knees would feel so much better."

Weight loss reduces the stress on your knees, limits further injury, increases mobility, and reduces the risk of associated health problems. I know it is not easy to lose weight. And if you simply starve yourself and don't exercise, your body will go into hibernation mode, making it *more* difficult for you to lose weight. At my practice, we can help you find a good, nutritional diet and exercise program to help you achieve your goal.

Although anti-inflammatory medication does help decrease inflammation in the joint, why not try an anti-inflammatory diet? Sugar and processed foods cause inflammation of the arteries, contributing to heart disease, as well as inflammation of the joints, contributing to arthritis.[26] An anti-inflammatory diet can help you avoid having to take anti-inflammatory medication.

Just look at what it did for Mia, a forty-five-year-old administrative assistant who had been asking me for years to replace her knees. I told her she was too young and if she lost some weight, her knees would feel better. Not believing me, she went to a university center for a second opinion and was scheduled for surgery without hesitation. However, the center was booked solid, so they scheduled her surgery three months out. During that time, Mia lost twenty pounds, and her knees stopped hurting. She canceled the surgery and has remained my patient ever since.

---

26   Vasanti S. Malik et al., "Sugar-Sweetened Berverages, Obesity, Type 2 Diabetes Mellitus, and Cardiovascular Disease Risk," *Circulation* 121, no. 11 (March 2010): 1356–1364, https://doi.org/10.1161/ CIRCULATIONAHA.109.876185

7. Improve your bone health.

Patients with arthritis and osteoporosis have more pain in their joints than patients with strong, healthy bones. Improving your bone health with increased calcium intake, daily vitamin D, and weight-bearing exercises can lessen the pain of arthritis.

Furthermore, if you do need a total joint replacement, studies show that total joint implants in patients with osteoporosis don't last as long as in patients with strong bones or who are on bone-strengthening medication.[27] Patients with osteoporosis have more revision surgeries due to loosening of the prostheses, so at Romano Orthopaedic Center, we recommend checking your bone density, if warranted. Building up your bone density will lessen your pain if you have arthritis and improve your chances of having a long-lasting joint replacement (see chapter six).

8. Injections.

If conservative therapy is not enough, knee injections may help. They are not a cure. They cannot rebuild your cartilage. But they can "buy time" so you may resume your normal activities in comfort while delaying the need for surgical intervention. Injections may last three months up to a year. There are three types of injections:

- **Cortisone** is a steroid that stops the inflammation in the joint and relieves pain. I do not like to give it to younger patients or to patients with a little arthritis because it may contribute to the further breakdown of cartilage. Steroids given frequently may be necessary in some patients with specific diseases, but in the long term can make you retain

---

27   Linda A. Russell, "Osteoporosis and orthopedic surgery: effect of bone health on total joint arthroplasty outcome," *Current Rheumatology Reports* 15, no. 11 (November 2013): 371, https://doi.org/10.1007/s11926-013-0371-x

water, weaken your bones, raise your blood sugar, cause cataracts, and have many other side effects. However, steroids in your knee joint, given four times a year, are usually safe.

- **Hyaluronic acid** is the naturally occurring gel that lubricates the knee joint. Coincidentally, it is also found in the coxcombs of roosters. Hyaluronic acid is deficient in arthritic knees. Injecting it into your knee can give you up to one year of relief. Because these injections are very expensive, Medicare and most insurance companies regulate its use. They only allow injections if cortisone injections have failed, and injections can be given no more than every six months. Injections can be given all at one time or spread out over several weeks. I have found that a series of five injections, spaced one week apart, will improve your pain better than a single injection. Receiving injections in six-month intervals manages your pain better than waiting until your pain is unbearable. Therefore, if the hyaluronic acid shots help, I recommend scheduling your next series of injections six months and one day after your last injection.

- **Platelet-rich plasma (PRP) and stem cells** are your own cells, which are injected into your joint to stimulate cartilage regrowth. (PRP comes from your concentrated blood, and stem cells come from your bone marrow.) A recent study found that in patients with osteoarthritis of the knee, PRP injections significantly relieved more pain and improved function more for up to one year compared to patients who had hyaluronic acid injections.[28] Yet, insurance companies still consider PRP injections experimental and refuse to pay for such treatments. In my practice, we have had good results from these injections and will consider them for certain patients in special situations where surgical correction is not a good option.

When you've tried all of these measures and they don't seem to work any longer, and you are not ready for a rocking chair and shawl, then surgery may be your best option. If surgery is necessary, rapid and successful recovery is possible by optimizing your physical and nutritional health before surgery; performing surgery with computer-assisted, patient-specific total joint instrumentation; and using an aggressive rehab program, like the ones we give our athletes (see chapter eight).

As I've mentioned, obtaining and maintaining strong health is important to get you through surgery, should you need it. But it's more important simply to keep you moving. The next chapter discusses how to do that.

---

28 Carlos Meheux et al., "Efficacy of Intra-articular Platelet-Rich Plasma Injections in Knee Osteoarthritis: A Systematic Review," *Arthroscopy: The Journal of Arthroscopic and Related Surgery* 32, no. 3 (March 2016): 495–505, https://doi.org/10.1016/j.arthro.2015.08.005

CHAPTER 6

BETTER BONES, BETTER OVERALL HEALTH

Shirley was a sixty-one-year-old cashier with a medical history of hypertension (high blood pressure) and diabetes. She didn't get much exercise, and her only calcium intake was the milk she drank in her coffee.

One day, while leaving work, she slipped in the parking lot and fell on her outstretched right arm—her dominant one. The fall left her in a lot of pain and with a deformed wrist.

She went to the ER, where X-rays showed an osteopenic, comminuted (splintered), markedly displaced, intra-articular, distal radial fracture. (See Figure 1.) Let's just say that she had a bad wrist fracture in soft bone. The fracture was in a lot of pieces, out of alignment, and went into the joint. She could not use her hand and had no feeling in her thumb and index and middle fingers, suggesting a median nerve (carpal tunnel) injury.

Because the fracture went into the joint and was markedly displaced, she needed surgery to fix the fracture and line up the joint so she would be able to use her wrist in the future, while also minimizing the risk of arthritis. Because there was also nerve injury, I took her to surgery that evening. I set the fracture and put a plate and screws in the radius. (See Figure 2.)

She had never had a bone density test before, so I had her tested; her score was very low, as was her vitamin D level. That meant she was at an extremely high risk for another fracture down the road. I immediately started her on a weekly megadose of vitamin D, and she increased the daily intake of calcium in her diet. She started on medication to increase her bone density, and she began a daily exercise routine.

At three weeks post-op, her fracture was healing nicely, so she started occupational therapy, and at six weeks post-op, she returned to work.

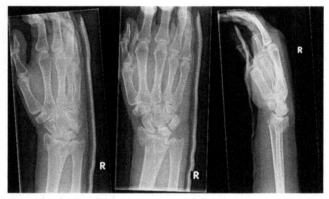

Fig. 1. X-ray of Shirley's fracture.

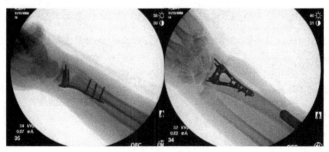

Fig. 2. Shirley's post-op X-rays.

Another case of mine was Peggy, a fifty-eight-year-old accountant who fell in her kitchen while preparing dinner. She broke her tibia (shinbone) and fibula. (See Figure 3.) The break left her bone protruding out of her skin. Her past medical history was significant in that she had a total hysterectomy (removal of her uterus and both ovaries) when she was thirty-five years old. Although patients with total hysterectomies at an early age are at increased risk of osteoporosis, she had never had a bone density exam, nor did she do anything to prevent bone loss.

Because her bone was exposed, she was at an extremely high risk for an infection, so I took her to surgery immediately for a washout of the fracture site and a repair of her tibia and fibula. (See Figure 4.)

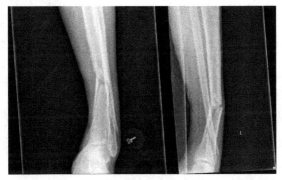

Fig. 3. X-rays of Peggy's fractures.

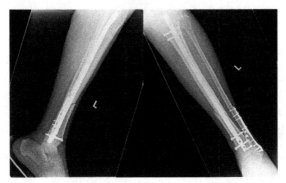

Fig. 4. Peggy's post-op X-rays after the fracture had healed.

The most pivotal bone case I ever have had was Mimi, an eighty-one-year-old who lived alone in a two-story home and used a walker when she left the house. In 2009, she had a right total hip replacement after a fall and fracture. In 2012, she had another fall and fractured her left hip, which also required surgical correction. She healed well after the second surgery. During her last visit, I told her that her bones were soft and she needed to see her primary care physician to get a bone density exam and be treated for osteoporosis. I also recommended she move out of her home and into a one-story condo.

She didn't follow any of my advice. Less than one year later, she returned to the ER with a new right femur fracture below the total hip prosthesis that had been inserted after her first fracture. (See Figure 5.) While doing laundry in her basement, she twisted to put clothes in the dryer, felt a snap in her right leg, and fell to the ground. Unable to walk to reach the phone, she lay on the basement floor until her daughter found her two days later.

After I repaired her leg, she spent four days in the ICU, a week in the hospital, and another three weeks in rehab. (See Figure 6.) She was lucky to recover quite well. She moved into the first floor of her daughter's home until she could move into an assisted living facility.

After that, I told her she no longer needed a bone density exam to diagnose her osteoporosis. She had proven it many times over. Then and there, I decided to take over all care for her bones and all of my patients' bones. Mimi was the first patient in the Romano Bone Health Clinic. After speaking to her primary care physician, I started her on daily injections she administered on her own for two years to increase her bone density. Now she is on twice-a-year injections to maintain her improved bone density. I also make sure she gets bone density exams every two years. In those appointments, I talk to her about her nutrition and getting enough calcium in her diet. I also monitor her vitamin D level and her bone health labs. I check her balance and encourage her to routinely exercise to help maintain her core strength. Today, I am happy to report she hasn't suffered any new fractures.

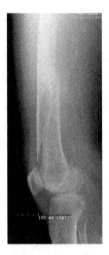

Fig. 5. Mimi's femur fracture below the nail.

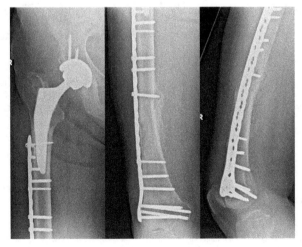

Fig. 6. X-rays of Mimi's repaired femur.

These cases all have one thing in common: The patient fell from a standing height and broke a bone. Normally, when you fall from a standing height, you don't expect to hurt yourself too seriously. When you fall from a standing height and break a bone, that's a problem.

Falls are the leading cause of death from injury in Americans over the age of sixty-five.[29]

Falls from a standing height are called *fragility fractures*. Over the last twenty-five years, I've seen a lot of fragility fractures. They are very painful and disruptive to life. The worst are hip fractures. Every year, I personally treat about twenty-five to fifty hip fractures. Older, sicker people get hip fractures more easily, and letting them go without corrective surgery is not an option. A patient with a fractured hip can't get up and go to the bathroom; they can't sit up and eat. They can easily get bedsores, blood clots, and pneumonia.

The statistics for hip fractures are pretty devastating. Within one year of falling and fracturing a hip, 20 percent of patients over age sixty-five die, 20 percent end up in a nursing home, and 30 percent drop one level in their walking ability.[30] This means if they didn't need an assistive device to walk before a hip fracture, afterwards they need a cane. If they already needed a cane, afterwards they need a walker. And if they previously needed a walker, afterwards they are only able to transfer in and out of a wheelchair. Only 30 percent of people over sixty-five are able to retain their same level of walking after a hip fracture.[31]

---

29   "Falls are leading cause of injury and death in older Americans," Centers of Disease Control and Prevention, September 22, 2016, https://www.cdc.gov/media/releases/2016/p0922-older-adult-falls.html.

30   Scott Schnell et al., "The 1-Year Mortality of Patients Treated in a Hip Fracture Program for Elders," *Geriatric Orthopaedic Surgery & Rehabilitation* 1, no. 1 (September 2010): 6–14, https://doi.org/10.1177/2151458510378105

I am passionate about properly treating osteoporosis. Doing so after an initial fragility fracture reduces the chance of having a second hip fracture by 25 to 50 percent.[32] Better yet, preventing osteoporosis in the first place can help avoid a broken arm or hip from a simple fall. You'll be a lot better off, and I'll be able to spend more time with my family—including my granddaughters, Mia and Ava.

WHAT IS OSTEOPOROSIS?

Osteoporosis is a serious bone disease that occurs when you lose too much bone, make too little bone, or both. It progresses without symptoms or pain. As a result, bones become thin and weak and can break easily.

There are a number of symptoms that may indicate thinning bones. In the elderly, these include back pain and loss of height. My dad was five-foot-six most of his life. But by the time he was eighty years old, he had shrunk to five-foot-two inches. This is because, with osteoporosis, the vertebrae weaken and collapse, causing the body to shrink. That also can cause curvature of the spine, back pain, and even trouble breathing. Unfortunately, many people are unaware they have osteoporosis until they suffer a fragility fracture. That's why whenever I see someone for the first time for any injury or complaint, I assess their bone health. My goal is to provide comprehensive, leading-edge care, from prevention to diagnosis and treatment.

---

31 Naoshi Fukui et al., "Predictors for ambulatory ability and the change in ADL after hip fracture in patients with different levels of mobility before injury: a 1-year prospective cohort study," *Journal of Orthopaedic Trauma* 26, no. 3 (March 2012): 163–71, https://doi.org/10.1097/BOT.0b013e31821e1261

32 Richard M. Dell et al., "Osteoporosis Disease Management: What Every Orthopaedic Surgeon Should Know," *Journal of Bone and Joint Surgery* 91, no. 6 (November 2009) :79–86, https://doi.org/10.2106/JBJS.I.00521

RISK FACTORS FOR OSTEOPOROSIS

- You are a female over sixty-five or a male over seventy.
- You've suffered a fracture from a standing height.
- You've lost 2 cm or more in height.
- You've been taking steroids for an extended time.
- You live an inactive lifestyle (fewer than 2.5 hours of exercise weekly).
- A family member has had osteoporosis or a hip fracture.
- You are a smoker or have more than two alcoholic beverages per day.
- You are not getting enough calcium or vitamin D in your diet.

TESTS FOR OSTEOPOROSIS

Bone density scans, also called dual-energy X-ray absorptiometry (DEXA) scans, are the only tests that can diagnose osteoporosis before a person breaks a bone. (See Figure 8.) Essentially, they are standardized X-rays of the spine and wrist that compare the patient's bone density to that of a healthy twenty-year-old. The result of the test is a "t-score." A bone density t-score between –1 and –2.5 (i.e., 1 to 2.5 standard deviations below a twenty-year-old's bone density) indicates osteopenia, or low bone density. A t-score below –2.5 indicates osteoporosis.

FRAX, a fracture risk assessment tool available online and developed at the University of Sheffield, calculates the ten-year probability of having a major osteoporotic fracture in the spine, forearm, hip, or shoulder.[33] (See Figure 9.) The scores are based on the

---

33 "FRAX, Fracture Risk Assessment Tool," Centre for Metabolic Bone Diseases, University of Sheffield, UK, accessed October 15, 2017, https://www.sheffield.ac.uk/FRAX/tool.jsp.

patient's birth country, age, sex, weight, height, previous fractures, parents' history of hip fracture, smoking, steroid treatment, rheumatoid arthritis, diseases strongly associated with osteoporosis, alcohol intake, and bone density t-score.

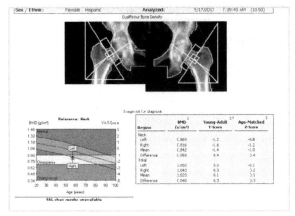

Fig. 8. DEXA scan results.

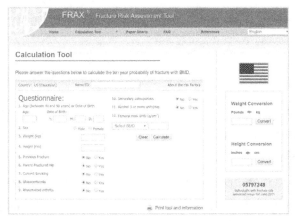

Fig. 9. Online FRAX calculator

TREATMENT FOR BETTER BONES

To prevent osteoporotic bone fractures, the US National Osteoporosis Foundation recommends treatment for osteoporosis for postmenopausal women and men older than fifty years of age if any of the following are present:

1. Prior hip or vertebral fracture

2. T-score of −2.5 at the femoral neck or spine, excluding secondary causes

3. T-score between −1.0 and −2.5 at the femoral neck or spine *and* a 10-year probability of hip fracture ≥ 3 percent *or* a 10-year probability of any other major osteoporotic fracture ≥ 20 percent

A clinician's judgment, in combination with patient preferences, may indicate treatment for people with ten-year fracture probabilities above or below these levels.[34]

Medication

Medication to help strengthen bones includes hormone replacement therapy for women experiencing early menopause or who have had a hysterectomy.

Bisphosphonates taken daily, weekly, monthly, or semiannually can slow or prevent bone loss and strengthen bones. Bisphosphonates inhibit the formation of osteoclasts, which are cells that are part of the remodeling process bones constantly undergo. Osteoclasts break down bone, while osteoblasts (other cells) rebuild bone. These two

---

34 F. Cosman et al., "Clinician's Guide to Prevention and Treatment of Osteoporosis," *Osteoporosis International* 25, no. 10 (August 2014): 2359–2381, https://doi.org/10.1007/s00198-014-2794-2

types of cells are typically in equilibrium, but fewer osteoclasts lead to an increase in bone mass.

Prolia is an injection administered semiannually to help women with postmenopausal osteoporosis strengthen their bones to reduce the risk of fracture. It is also used to treat bone loss in men and women receiving certain cancer drugs that increase the risk for fractures.

The only medication that directly promotes the buildup of bone is parathyroid hormones, which can be self-injected daily for eighteen months to two years. Although studies in rats using high doses of parathyroid hormones for an extended period of time show an increase in bone cancer, there hasn't been a problem in humans using a low dose for two years or less.[35]

Diet and Nutrition

The best way to strengthen your bones is to increase your daily intake of calcium and vitamin D.

Calcium is a mineral used for building and maintaining strong bones and teeth. Not made in the body, calcium must be absorbed from the foods you eat and is stored in your bones. However, the body can only store calcium in the bones during youth—until age twenty-one in males and twenty-six in females. It's like depositing money in the bank. The less calcium taken in when you're young, the less calcium stored in your bones for the rest of your life. So, at maturity, your bones are as strong as they will get. Bone strength can only decrease with age.

Calcium is also essential for proper functioning of the heart, brain, and nerves. Adults need about 1,200 mg of calcium per day. A diet low in calcium will cause the body to steal the mineral away

---

35 Stephanie K.A. Blick, Sohita Dhillon, and Susan J. Keam, "Teriparatide: A Review of its Use in Osteoporosis," *Drugs* 68, no. 18 (2008): 2709–37, https://doi-org.mwu.idm.oclc.org/10.2165/0003495-200868180-00012

from the bones to maintain normal blood calcium levels. Over time, this leads to weaker bones and, eventually, fragility fractures.

It's important to note your body will only absorb up to 1,500 mg of calcium per day. So trying to "overload" on calcium to "make up for some lost time" is ineffective, results in high calcium levels in the urine and stool, and increases the risk of constipation and/or kidney stones.

I recommend getting calcium from your diet rather than in pill form. Some studies argue taking high doses of calcium in pill form may increase the risk of heart attacks and strokes. It is believed in pill form, calcium is absorbed too rapidly. When the calcium blood level spikes, calcium sticks to the plaque in the blood vessels, increasing the chance of heart attacks and strokes. Calcium in food form is absorbed more slowly, thereby decreasing the chance of sticking to plaque and may even lower the risk of coronary artery disease.[36] However, other studies refute this theory.[37] Regardless, if you don't get enough calcium from your diet, take no more than 500 mg of calcium in pill form at one time. Choose calcium citrate for better absorption, and ensure it contains vitamin D.

36   John J.B. Anderson et al., "Calcium Intake From Diet and Supplements and the Risk of Coronary Artery Calcification and its Progression Among Older Adults: 10-Year Follow-up of the Multi-Ethnic Study of Atherosclerosis (MESA)," Journal of the American Heart Association 5, no.10 (October 2016), https://doi.org/10.1161/JAHA.116.003815

37   Joshua R. Lewis, "Calcium supplementation and the risks of atherosclerotic vascular disease in older women: Results of a 5-year RCT and a 4.5-year follow-up," Journal of Bone and Mineral Research 26, no.1 (January 2011): 35-41, https://doi.org/10.1002/jbmr.176

WAYS TO ADD CALCIUM TO YOUR DIET

- Start your day with calcium-fortified orange juice.

- Cook cereals with skim milk or almond milk (instead of water), or add two tablespoons of nonfat dry milk.

- Drink low-fat or fat-free milk with meals. (If you are lactose intolerant, try lactose-free milk or almond milk.)

- Spread low-fat cream cheese on bread or toast instead of butter or margarine.

- Add low-fat cheeses to sandwiches, salads, and pizzas.

- Add sardines to salads or sandwiches.

- Include higher-calcium greens such as spinach, broccoli, and kale in your salad.

- Enjoy low-fat or fat-free yogurt with berries for dessert.

- Make smoothies with frozen fruit, fortified orange juice, and low-fat or fat-free yogurt.

Vitamin D is important for the absorption of calcium and aids in improving muscle strength and balance. Vitamin D deficiency also is associated with depression, Parkinson's disease, and seizures. It is estimated that 10 percent of the American population is vitamin D deficient. A recent study has shown that up to 50 percent of patients who were seen in an orthopaedic trauma center were vitamin D deficient.[38] And it's worse where I'm located, in Chicago, because sunshine is the best source of vitamin D, and we have fewer sunny days than most other major cities in the United States.

In my office, 80 percent of patients with fractures are vitamin D deficient, so I start them on a prescription dose of vitamin D. The

---

38   Barbara Steele et al., "Vitamin D Deficiency: A Common Occurrence in Both High-and Low-energy Fractures," *HSS Journal* 4, no.2 (September 2008): 143–148, https://doi.org/10.1007/s11420-008-9083-6

FDA's official dietary recommendations are 600 IU daily until age seventy and 800 IU after that.[39] Many experts believe these recommendations are far too low to maintain healthy vitamin D levels. Research also shows that consuming 1,000 IU daily would help 50 percent of people reach a normal vitamin D blood level. Consuming 2000 IU daily would help nearly everyone reach a normal blood level.[40] Taking up to 10,000 IU of vitamin D a day is safe, but don't do that without a doctor's recommendation.[41] Vitamin D3 is the best form of vitamin D to take.

Again, sunshine is considered the best source for vitamin D, and ten minutes a day will do it—depending on where you're located. In July in Cape Cod, for instance, fifteen minutes in the sun in shorts and a T-shirt delivers 10,000 IU. But north of Atlanta, the sun is not high enough from October to May to produce enough vitamin D. In Chicago, as I mentioned, where there are eighty-five sunny days a year (versus 275 in Las Vegas), vitamin D deficiency is more prevalent. In spite of what dermatologists warn, spend ten minutes in the sun and then put on sunscreen and a hat—and if necessary, take vitamin D!

39 "Vitamin D Fact Sheet for Consumers," National Institutes of Health, April 15, 2016, https://ods.od.nih.gov/factsheets/VitaminD-Consumer.

40 Reinhold Vieth et al., "The urgent need to recommend an intake of vitamin D that is effective," *The American Journal of Clinical Nutrition* 85, no. 3 (March 2007): 649–650, http://ajcn.nutrition.org/content/85/3/649.full

41 John N. Hathcock et al., "Risk assessment for vitamin D," *The American Journal of Clinical Nutrition* 85, no.1 (January 2007): 6-18, http://ajcn.nutrition.org/content/85/1/6.full

PREVENTING OSTEOPOROSIS AND FRAGILITY FRACTURES

Besides medication and dietary supplements, there are many other ways to prevent osteoporosis and fragility fractures naturally. These include:

Get ample exercise.

Every day, incorporate weight-bearing activities into your routine. These can help preserve bone density and maintain muscle strength. Consider activities like weight training, walking, hiking, running, elliptical, stationary bike, or even dancing. Resistive exercises, including working out with bands, push-ups, and pull-ups, also can help. Physical therapy, including using a vibrating plate, is another way to stimulate bone strength.

Prevent falls.

Preventing falls inside and outside the home can help prevent fragility fractures.

Inside the home, keep the floors smooth (but not slippery) and clear of clutter. Don't walk around in socks or floppy slippers. Use no-slip rugs on floors and rubber mats in the shower or tub. Install railings on both sides of the stairs and in the shower and tub. Use nightlights. Move the washer and dryer out of the basement.

Outside the home, take care with curbs before stepping up or down. Watch out for potholes in streets and sidewalks. Use the railings on stairs. In wet weather, take extra care to avoid slipping in water on the ground. In winter, wear shoes with good traction and coats with adequate padding. And in bad weather, ask for help or consider using a cane or walker. (People are nicer to you when you have a cane.)

In addition, tai chi, swimming, and stretching exercises can improve your balance and prevent falls.

Don't smoke!

Besides causing heart and lung disease, smoking is toxic to bones and can lead to osteoporosis and fragility fractures. If you do get a fracture, smoking will delay healing and increase the risk of deep vein thrombosis (a blood clot) and stroke after a fracture. It also increases the risk of complications after surgery such as infections, pneumonia, heart attacks, and death.

Limit alcohol intake.

Heavy drinking can increase bone loss and increase the risk of fracture after a fall. The National Osteoporosis Foundation states that consuming three or more alcoholic drinks per day is detrimental to your health.

Eat a well-balanced, healthy diet.

Read food labels and choose foods and beverages high in calcium and vitamin D. Avoid sodas, as the phosphates in soda bind to and deplete calcium. Look for calcium-fortified foods (foods that do not normally contain calcium but have added calcium). Examples include fortified orange juice and ready-to-eat cereals.

Get some sun.

A mere ten to fifteen minutes of sunlight at least three times per week can dramatically improve your bone health.

These measures can help reduce your risk for a fracture and keep you from needing surgery.

In the next chapter, I'll discuss nonsurgical fixes for other types of common injuries.

CHAPTER 7

NONSURGICAL TREATMENTS FOR SPORTS AND OTHER INJURIES

As a team physician, I've been on the sidelines of games since my first year in medical school. Once I learned AMNRT testing, I couldn't wait to test it on our football players. The only problem was that there was only one of me. I couldn't test all the players all the time.

During the 2015 season, we had a great team and hoped to make it to the state final. Unfortunately, we lost early on in the playoffs. The problem was losing seven players to season-ending injuries. When I examined each player after their injury, I found at least one positive reflex. I wished I would have known about AMNRT beforehand; perhaps their injuries could have been avoided.

The following season, I treated all players like they already had an injury. I demonstrated my balance testing to the team, starting with the biggest and toughest players. When I was able to knock guys twice my size off-balance, I had the team's attention.

After that, I showed them how to do my "Romano Stretches" to reverse existing problems and help protect them against injury. That season, they all did the stretches before every practice, before every game, and at halftime of every game. We had our best season in years.

A controversial call ultimately kept our team from going to the state championship, but more importantly, we finished the season with the same players with whom we started. Incredibly, only two players missed a total of five games all season long due to injuries during play.

Seeing the success with the football team, I decided to use AMNRT and Romano stretches with the school's hockey and basketball teams. Both teams finished second in state, with only one player on the basketball team missing a game because of tendinitis (he didn't do his stretches), two suffering from concussions, and one on the hockey team suffering a spine fracture—the result of being slammed into the boards (he's fine now).

As I've mentioned, finding the source of pain can help cure a problem using nonsurgical means and it can change someone's life.

Lizzie is a good example of that. She is an extremely competitive, energetic, fifty-four-year-old, dot-com executive and avid tennis player who travels the country for work and to play tennis. She first came to see me for tennis elbow in her right arm. Multiple injections by other doctors, several tennis elbow bands, medication, extensive physical therapy, and expensive trainers had not provided her much relief. Lizzie was one of the best players on her traveling team but had become unable to participate in a national championship tennis tournament, so she wanted surgery.

No question, she did have tennis elbow; however, using AMNRT, I found bilateral CTS, right cubital tunnel syndrome, right TMD, left sacroiliitis (inflammation where the spine and pelvis connect), obstructed breathing, and sleep apnea. She did not offer up any of these problems in her history. When I asked her about the numbness in her hands, she was a little surprised. She said, "Oh, that only happened a few times. It doesn't bother me. What about my elbow?" As I noted in an earlier chapter, pain in one area of the body is often associated with an injury on the other side of the body. For instance, TMD on the right side of the face is always associated with left sacroiliitis; it's a reflex. Left sacroiliitis is always associated with weakness in the opposite elbow—another reflex. When I asked her about her back pain, she said, "How did you know?" She had been bothered by back pain most of her adult life. She simply lived with it. Therapy, massages, constant stretching, pain meds including narcotics, and acupuncture helped. Surprisingly, she never realized her elbow was weaker. It just always hurt.

I also noticed her tongue was scalloped. I asked her about her sleeping habits and if she grinded her teeth at night. Those questions actually made her a little nervous—she wasn't sure why an orthopaedist was asking her so many personal details. She told me she woke up once or twice a night to go to the bathroom. "So what? I drink a lot of water. But sleeping is not a problem, I take sleeping pills," she said. I was fairly certain a sleep test would show she had sleep apnea. But instead of finding out why she wasn't sleeping well, her doctors had prescribed sleeping pills.

Finally, I asked her about her stomach pain and diarrhea. Since she hadn't mentioned those as symptoms, she was truly shocked to hear me ask about them. I explained it was impossible to have all the problems she was experiencing without her gut responding negatively because her body was in dystrophy. Her sympathetic system was in overdrive. But she had stopped complaining about stomach pain and diarrhea a long time ago because nothing her doctor did helped. That made her cry; despite her outgoing personality, she revealed she was chronically depressed—something she also took pills for.

Lizzie was going to need more than just stretching to turn around all of her health problems, but her condition was already improving just by finding a provider who could help her get to the root of her problems and address them with nonsurgical solutions.

TREATMENT WITHOUT SURGERY

The treatment for most musculoskeletal injuries is rest, ice, compression, and elevation (RICE).

Rest. If a part of your body hurts, it's telling you to stop! "Don't keep aggravating me, or I'll make you pay for it later." Listen to your body.

Ice, compression, and elevation of a body part helps limit swelling. Ice is the best anti-inflammatory. Try twenty minutes on and twenty minutes off for an hour or two. Don't leave the ice on for more than twenty minutes at a time, otherwise you may get frostbite and blisters. (Trust me. I've done it myself before. Oops!) Try massaging the ice for five to ten minutes directly over the injured area. When you wrap an extremity, don't make it too tight. You can cut off the circulation.

You also can try over-the-counter NSAIDs to prevent or decrease inflammation. Read the labels for dosage directions to avoid burning a hole in your stomach or causing internal bleeding.

Here is a list of the top ten sports injuries I see often that can be treated without surgery.

#1: Shoulder Pain

Although it's the body's weakest joint, the shoulder is subject to a great deal of force during athletic activities. It is no wonder shoulder injuries are common in overhead sports. The rotator cuff and scapular (shoulder blade or wing bone) stabilizing muscles hold the shoulder in place as it goes through its wide range of motion. If these muscles are weak, the shoulder tends to slouch forward and impinges on the acromion (part of the scapular bone that sits above the rotator cuff), causing pain, swelling, and instability.

Treatment with RICE and anti-inflammatories will resolve the symptoms, but if you don't strengthen the muscles to bring the shoulder back in place and keep it in place, the problem and pain will return. Therapy consists of scapular stabilizing exercises to bring the shoulders back. These include front, overhead, and upward pulls and reverse flies.

But it isn't always that easy. Despite extensive rehab, the pain sometimes persists, even when an MRI does not show a tear. That's when I look for other sources. When pain goes down the arm to the elbow and hand, I usually find carpal and/or cubital tunnel syndromes associated with the pain. Stretching and avoiding certain activities help resolve the issue. (See the sections on carpal and cubital tunnel syndromes in chapter two.)

If the shoulder pain starts from or goes between the scapulae, then it may be associated with posterior rib subluxation (see chapter two).

When shoulder weakness and neck and/or back pain accompany shoulder pain, I look for neck and back problems associated with obstructive breathing disorder (see chapter three). Remember, when someone's breathing is obstructed, their airway opens more when their head is tilted forward and the shoulders follow. So, no matter how strong the shoulder muscles are, if an athlete or anyone has obstructed breathing, he or she will not keep the shoulders back indefinitely. Breathing will always win out, and the head and shoulders will begin to slouch forward to keep the airway open. Therefore, it is imperative to fix the source of the problem by correcting the breathing. Furthermore, if pain is worse at night, sleep apnea is a suspect.

Finally, when the pain is associated with loss of motion, especially loss of internal rotation, pelvic tilt may be an aggravating problem (see chapter four). Lower back stretches and a pelvic stabilizing program will help.

#2 Tennis Elbow

Tennis elbow, or lateral epicondylitis, is typically associated with pain and burning on the outer elbow (the lateral epicondyle) and is aggravated by gripping and lifting with the wrist. Holding a tennis racket, shaking hands, lifting a suitcase, and turning a doorknob can be painful. The mechanism of injury is tearing of the muscle attached to the lateral epicondyle that lifts the wrist. Typically, this injury comes from repetitive use.

The first course of treatment is RICE. You can use a tennis elbow splint for counter compression (limiting the muscle pull on the elbow) along with a wrist brace to keep the wrist stable, so you don't have to use the muscle when using the hand. Therapy includes muscle stretching and strengthening with eccentric (exercises that lengthen the muscle with increasing intensity) and progressive resistive exercises. Modalities such as an ultrasound and cold laser treatment can help recondition the tendon.

Before having surgery to release the attachment of the muscle from the elbow to remove the strain, try an elbow injection. A cortisone injection will decrease the inflammation at the elbow, allowing the muscle to heal. If that doesn't work, a PRP injection can help. Medical insurance and workers' comp insurances usually will approve a PRP injection if all other conservative treatment fails to work. It's cheaper and less painful than surgery.

That is the typical approach I've used for years to treat tennis elbow. With AMNRT, I have learned it is far better, and with longer lasting results, to get to the source of tennis elbow. Why are you using more force on that elbow for gripping or lifting? AMNRT may reveal the hand is weak from carpal and/or cubital tunnel syndromes you most likely never realized you have. Or, if you do realize it, the pain and tingling are only an annoyance—nothing like the tennis elbow pain. Nevertheless, if your hand is weak, you will require considerably more force to use your hand and wrist, resulting in microtears of the wrist muscle attachment at the elbow. Fix the carpal and cubital tunnel problems, and your elbow pain will begin to heal on its own. (See the sections on carpal and cubital tunnel in chapter two.)

#3 Groin Pain

Pain in the groin can be related to a strain of the inner thigh muscles (adductors or hip flexors), a labral tear, or a sports hernia. Common symptoms include pain when climbing stairs, getting in and out of a car, or quickly moving from side to side.

Common causes are sprinting, running inclines, and sudden starts or changes in direction while playing sports.

As with most injuries, RICE and NSAIDs are helpful, as are gentle stretches. Physical therapy for specific hip-strengthening exercises can help you regain power, range of motion, and movement more quickly. AMNRT may reveal a sports hernia. If so, a simple stretching and strengthening program may alleviate your symptoms. (See chapter two.)

Proper stretching before and after exercise, as well as avoiding strenuous exercise while fatigued, may prevent straining a groin muscle. Gradually increasing the intensity of your workout, rather than jumping in too quickly, can also help avoid groin pain.

A catching or locking sensation in the groin or a severe, intermittent, sharp pain with activity may indicate a labral tear. If the pain persists, an MRI can confirm the diagnosis of a labral tear.

One patient, a thirty-five-year-old engineer, came to see me for a hip arthroscopy to fix a questionable labral tear seen on his hip MRI. He could not play soccer because of groin pain that had started months prior. While shoveling snow, he twisted and immediately felt a sharp pain in his groin. On exam, the typical compression test for labral tear was negative, but his sports hernia reflex was positive. With a simple manipulation of the groin, his pain subsided. Within a week, he was playing soccer again and is still playing. He never did have a hip arthroscopy.

#4 Patellofemoral Symptoms

Patellofemoral pain syndrome, otherwise known as *chondromalacia patella* or *runner's knee*, is one of the most common problems I see in my office. Patients complain of vague pain around the kneecap with prolonged sitting, squatting, jumping, or stairclimbing (especially when going down). Occasionally, they experience knee buckling, or sudden giving way of the knee. Catching, popping, or grinding sensations while walking is also common. This injury is thought to come from overuse, injury, excess weight, poor alignment of the kneecap, or arthritis under the kneecap.

X-rays and MRIs are usually normal or show some wear under the kneecap. When the outside structures (iliotibial band and ligaments) are tight, and the inside muscle (vastus medialis oblique) is weak, the kneecap does not track well in its groove. Surgery, involving cutting the outside structures and tightening the inside ones, can correct the alignment but is only 50 percent successful. You don't want a surgery that is only as predictable as a coin toss. Therapy, stretching the outside structures and strengthening the inside muscles, are better solutions.

A patella knee sleeve with a hole in the middle and/or taping the kneecap will help keep the patella on track while undergoing therapy.

Wearing good shoes with arch supports will align the foot and, in turn, the knee, helping patellar tracking.

But what is the true source of patellofemoral pain? With patients who have patellofemoral pain in the right knee, I routinely find weakness in their right hip flexors, as well as unrecognized pain in their left feet. Their body is subconsciously protecting the left foot while placing more weight on the weak right leg, resulting in patellofemoral pain. The pain in the opposite foot—Morton's neuroma, and/or peroneal neuropathy—easily can be treated with proper stretching, supportive shoes, and avoiding forced hyperextension of the foot (see the sections on Morton's neuroma and peroneal neuropathy in chapter two). I have a little more difficulty convincing my patients that the source of their leg weakness is due to their lower back when it really doesn't bother them (see chapter three). They have even more difficulty believing me when I tell them their back problem is related to their obstructed breathing. Only when these issues are addressed will full healing occur.

#5 Shin Splints

Shin splints are pains on the inside of the lower leg bone, the tibia. They can be caused by running or jumping on hard surfaces, increasing workout intensity too quickly, wearing worn-out shoes, or simply overuse. Shin splints can progress to a stress fracture, which can be debilitating.

Typical treatment involves RICE and anti-inflammatories. Athletic shoes with good arch supports, stretching, changing running surfaces from asphalt to grass or a running track, and a more gradual increase in running activities will help prevent recurrence.

Using AMNRT, I usually find patients with shin splints have Morton's neuroma and peroneal neuropathy on the same and/or opposite foot. When I check their vitamin D level, I usually find it low, so stretching the feet and increasing daily vitamin D and calcium intake will address the source of the pain and speed recovery.

#6 Achilles Tendinitis

The largest tendon in the body, the Achilles tendon, is in the back of the ankle. Achilles tendinitis is the inflammation of this tendon; it is most common in athletes participating in running and jumping activities. Excessive pronation of the foot (flatfoot) can aggravate the problem. If left untreated, Achilles tendinitis can become chronic, making it difficult to run.

Treatment includes RICE and NSAIDs. Over-the-counter or custom arch supports are often necessary to correct excessive pronation. Stretching and strengthening exercises for the calf muscles can help heal Achilles tendinitis and prevent further injuries.

If you have Achilles tendinitis, remember to look for and treat Morton's neuroma and peroneal neuropathy in the same and/ or opposite foot. They can be the source of your problem. (See chapter two.)

#7 Ankle Sprain

Ankle sprains are very common among athletes competing in running and jumping sports, and any sport involving cutting maneuvers (football, soccer, etc). A **mild** ankle injury occurs when an athlete gently twists his or her ankle and stretches the ligaments. No real tearing occurs. A **moderate** ankle sprain occurs with a little more force when an athlete lunges over a poorly planted foot and partially tears the ligaments. A **severe** ankle injury occurs after forcefully twisting the foot while running or jumping, tearing the ligaments completely. A general rule of thumb is that an X-ray is needed only if you cannot walk on the injured ankle.

Treatment includes RICE and NSAIDs, ankle braces, and walking boots. Keep your ankle iced and elevated as soon as possible after an injury. Do not allow it to swell. The more it swells, the longer it will take to heal. But don't immobilize it for too long. Gentle, early range-of-motion stretches improve circulation and will allow you to return to sports sooner. To do this, "write the alphabet" with your foot, gradually increasing the size of the lettering.

Single-legged toe raises are excellent balance and strengthening exercises for the ankle. I also recommend taping the ankle or wearing a lace-up brace for at least three months after an injury to prevent recurrence.

Again, you should look for and treat Morton's neuroma and peroneal neuropathy of the opposite foot (see chapter two). Furthermore, if you have either injury, your balance is off, and you will be more prone to falling; when you misstep, your body will subconsciously protect your hurt foot, and you will end up injuring the opposite foot instead.

#8 Plantar Fasciitis

Plantar fasciitis is heel pain at the bottom of the foot, usually with the first morning steps. The pain is thought to be from microtears of the ligament attached to the heel. Within the first few weeks, rest, activity modification, and stretching may be all that is needed. Over-the-counter arch supports, custom orthotics, splinting, and injections also may help. Surgery is only the last resort and is rarely necessary. Correcting Morton's neuroma on the same or opposite foot will help alleviate the heel pain and prevent a recurrence. (See chapter two.)

#9 Sciatica

Sciatica affects up to 40 percent of people at some point in their life. Characterized by pain in the lower back going down the leg, it usually is attributed to a herniated disc or spinal arthritis pushing on the spinal nerve roots. I have found that pelvic tilting, Morton's neuroma, peroneal nerve entrapment, and obstructed breathing (with its associated back problems) all aggravate sciatica symptoms. Accurately diagnosing and treating these sources will significantly relieve symptoms. And if you are waking up with severe lower back pain at night, sleep apnea, with its drop in blood oxygen levels from not breathing, may be contributing to your pain.

#10 Concussions

When I was in school playing sports, I thought I was indestructible. Whenever I "had my bell rung" (and I did, multiple times), I just would shake it off and get back on the field or in the ring. But that's not healthy. A concussion is a brain injury—that's serious! Once your brain is injured and before it is completely healed, you are more susceptible to another, more devastating injury called *second impact syndrome.* A second blow to the head, even a minor hit, can cause the brain to swell, leading to coma and death. Concussions also can lead to a host of symptoms: post-concussion syndrome, depression, tiredness, inability to concentrate, chronic traumatic encephalopathy, and more.

I am very serious about concussions when it comes to the athletes I help. I can take care of sprains easily—a splint will help you heal and keep you safe, and you'll be back on the field pretty quickly. But that doesn't work with head injuries.

At the beginning of every school year, before they can put on a uniform, our student athletes take a baseline computerized concussion test. During a practice or game, if a concussion even is suspected, they are finished playing for that day immediately. Period. Just as we rest their ankle after an ankle sprain, we rest their brain after a concussion. They do not return to play until they are completely symptom-free, return to the baseline computerized test score, and successfully complete a sport-specific, five-day, return-to-play protocol. Their teachers all get a note excusing them from or postponing homework, papers, and tests. They even may receive a program that reads to them, or they will have an assistant read to them, if necessary.

Over the years, there have been several players who have had prolonged post-concussion symptoms, sometimes lasting longer than one month. Formal vestibular training (a balance rehab protocol) has been helpful in restoring their balance. However, I have found that athletes with prolonged symptoms also have positive AMNRT reflexes with the corresponding loss of balance. Before the concussion, the athletes were able to compensate for this balance problem without much trouble. However, after the concussion, they lose their ability to compensate, and their balance is way off. Reversing the AMNRT reflexes after a concussion—or better yet, before a concussion—restores balance better and quicker than vestibular retraining. This gets our athletes and others suffering from concussions back on the field or back to daily living a little easier, a little faster, and a lot safer.

So again, there are ways to address injuries without surgery, but there are also injuries and instances when surgical intervention is absolutely necessary, as I will describe for you in the next chapter.

CHAPTER 8
SURGERY—WHEN IT'S RIGHT

My mother was eighty-three when she had her hip replaced. (I did not perform the surgery.) While wintering in Florida, Mom would walk two miles every day to the Four Seasons Hotel, read their newspaper, drink their coffee, and then walk home. When she had to give all that up because of hip pain, she wanted a total hip replacement, and she wanted it yesterday. She came through the surgery and recovery just fine.

One year later, Mom's knee was her limiting factor, so she also had a total knee replacement on the opposite leg of her hip replacement. Now, at age eighty-six, Mom gives me a daily report of her activities. She walks 10,000 to 15,000 steps a day (her record is 27,000 steps during a recent trip to Rome). One of my younger total joint patients admonished me when I wasn't impressed he walked one mile, saying, "Stop comparing me to your mother."

As one of my nonagenarian patients once told me, "Never give up anything. Once you do, you never get it back." Never give up anything you enjoy doing. My dad was an avid golfer, so my number one rule is that if your injury is preventing you from playing golf or participating in anything else you enjoy doing, and conservative care has been unsuccessful, it's time for surgery.

There is a right time to have surgery.

My grandmother was eighty-five when I was an orthopaedic resident and suggested she have a total knee replacement. She was ready to do so, but everyone else talked her out of it, saying she was "too old" and "would never do the rehab." She lived to be ninety-four, but without a knee replacement, her final years were racked with pain. It upset her that she could only make one apple pie because her knees were too painful to make two. It pained me to hear her say, "I wish my mind would go, then I wouldn't care about my knees."

There's a window of opportunity to have a joint replacement. In her nineties, Grama's heart would not have withstood the surgery, but at eighty-five, she was in good health and would have done well with surgery.

"There are two types of retirement," a patient once told me, "active retirement and rocking chair retirement."

One day, Willard, a pleasant, ninety-year-old gentleman showed up at my office in the middle of the day to tell me he knew my grandfather. During the Great Depression, my grandfather treated Willard's mother after she severely burned herself while cooking. In return, she had paid him with chickens.

Willard originally had an appointment to see me, but his primary care physician told him to cancel it because he was too old for a knee replacement. At age ninety, Willard still worked in the forestry department, where he had worked for fifty-eight years. Until three months prior to seeing me, he had walked a mile to and from church each day, but he'd given that up because of his painful knees. He was in excellent health except for his knees, for which injections and arthritis medication had proved useless.

After examining Willard and talking to his doctor, I replaced his severely arthritic knee. He resumed walking to mass every day and finally retired from the forestry department on his sixtieth anniversary.

If you aren't ready for that rocking chair and shawl, and conservative care does not work, consider having your joints replaced.

TOP NINE SURGICAL PROCEDURES AND WHEN TO DO THEM

In my practice, I treat a wide range of orthopaedic health issues. Among these, here are the top nine problems that require surgical procedures.

#1 Total Joints

You know by now that I advocate conservative care as much as possible, but if conservative care worked 100 percent of the time, I would be out of a job! If you have debilitating pain and/or difficulty walking or climbing stairs because of severe degenerative arthritis despite the best conservative treatments, surgery is your best option no matter how old you are. Total hip and knee replacements are safe and effective in relieving pain, correcting deformities, and allowing you to resume normal activities. They can be truly life changing.

Once a decision is made, you need to see your primary care physician to ensure you are in the best possible health to have surgery. If you have any chronic medical conditions, like heart disease, you also should be evaluated by a relevant specialist, such as a cardiologist, before the surgery.

To best prepare for total joint surgery, we will give you this checklist of things to do:

- **See the dentist.** Although the risk of infection is low, if you have bleeding gums or an infected tooth, bacteria from your mouth can get into your bloodstream and infect the prosthesis site.

- **Get a bone density exam**. Patients with untreated osteoporosis have more fractures around and more loosening of total joint replacements. If you have osteoporosis, we will set you up with a treatment plan.

- **Screen for sleep apnea**. Patients with unrecognized or untreated sleep apnea have a 44 percent increase in postoperative complications.

- **Get pre-op tests**. Pre-op blood and urine tests assess nutritional health, diabetic control, anemia, underlying infections, and potential bleeding problems.

- **Adjust medications**. We will go over which medicines need to be adjusted before surgery and which medicines should be continued.

- **Make social arrangements**. If you live alone, you will need to plan for someone to assist you or plan to go to a rehab facility for a short stay.

- **Make home arrangements**. Simple modifications will make it safe for you to return home after surgery. These include safety bars in the shower or bath, handrails for stairs, raised toilet seats, a stable shower bench or chair, no loose carpets or cords, and a temporary living space downstairs until it is safe for you to go up and down stairs frequently.

Our hospital checklist includes pre-op antibiotics to prevent infections and anti-nausea medication to ensure you are comfortable after surgery.

The anesthesiologist administers a nerve block before the surgery to keep you comfortable after surgery. He or she will discuss the options of spinal or epidural anesthesia versus general, including the pros and cons of each. If you are healthy and have few or no medical issues, then general anesthesia is fine. If you have multiple medical conditions, such as heart issues and sleep apnea, they may recommend a spinal or epidural anesthesia. It is safer and requires much less anesthesia medication during surgery.

In general, the degenerative cartilage and surrounding bone of the knee are removed and replaced with metal and plastic. We use state-of-the-art instrumentation and computer-navigated guidance to measure the cuts to within 0.5 degrees and 0.5 millimeters. It's like playing a video game where everyone wins in the end.

After a short stay in the recovery room, where you will be monitored as you recover from anesthesia, you will be sent to the orthopaedic floor. Remember, while our team is extraordinary and extremely attentive to your needs, you are not in a luxury hotel where you will be pampered. I liken it more to the Notre Dame football boot camp, where they will work you hard to get you ready to be your best. On the same day as surgery, you'll be walking up and down the halls with one of the hospital therapists (I will even take you for a stroll after hours). Depending on your home status and your physical health, you will be in the hospital for one to two days and sent home with a visiting nurse and a home therapist. I do not believe in sending you home the same day as surgery unless you have a medical professional who is willing to wait on you around the clock—getting you up to the bathroom, dispensing your medications, monitoring your vital signs, checking for blood clots, and constantly assessing you for any other signs of problems. I do not feel it is safe for you or fair to your caregiver.

If you live by yourself or have no one who will be able to care for you in the days after surgery, you will be transferred to a rehab center for one to two weeks. You will be using a walker for a few days and then transition to a cane for a few more days—possibly up to two to three weeks. If your right knee is replaced, or as long as you are on narcotics, it is not safe to drive—usually for four to six weeks after surgery.

#2 Meniscus Tears

There are two types of cartilage in the knee: the articular cartilage, which covers the bones, and the meniscus, which cushions between the two bones. The consistency of the meniscus is like those large pink erasers you get in school. At the beginning of the school year, they're soft and malleable. You can bend and twist the rubber eraser without any problem. At the end of the school year, they are brittle and crumble when you bend or twist them. Fifty-year-old cartilage is like that eraser at the beginning of the second semester. When a person is in their twenties or thirties, it takes a significant sports injury to tear the meniscus. Over age fifty, just bend and twist the wrong way, and the meniscus tears.

When the meniscus tears, it rarely heals itself. Most of the time, it catches and locks between the two bones, damaging the articular cartilage and causing pain and swelling of the knee. When the articular cartilage wears down, that's when you get bone-on-bone arthritis.

If you're in your twenties and thirties and have a clean tear, it may be possible to save and repair the meniscus. That will leave the most cushioning in your knee. However, if you are older or have a chronic meniscus tear, the meniscus may be too shredded to be repaired and may have to be removed—but only the torn portion. The remaining meniscus is saved to maintain as much cushioning as possible.

Before knee arthroscopy was common, orthopaedists used to remove the entire meniscus, even for small tears. Their belief was that a patient didn't really need the meniscus; removing it would eliminate the need to come back for another surgery when it tore again. Some thought it would grow back. Both beliefs are wrong. You do need it, and the meniscus does not grow back. Those who had their meniscus completely removed in high school were looking at a knee replacement twenty years later. It is best to save the meniscus whenever possible. Although there is less than a 15 percent chance the repaired meniscus won't heal and another surgery will be needed to remove it, there's an 85 percent chance of never needing another surgery and having more cushioning for the rest of your life.[42]

When I scope the knee to fix the meniscus, I like to do it under local anesthesia with sedation. Patients can have as little or as much sedation as they choose. To me, the scariest thing about surgery is going to sleep. Why would you want someone to put a tube down your throat into your lungs to breathe for you when you could breathe on your own?

Before surgery, while you are in the pre-op holding area and adequately sedated, I give three shots of Novocain in the knee so it is numb by the time we start surgery. You will feel movement, and perhaps some stretching of your leg if the tear is way in the back, but you will feel no pain. If you want, you can watch your surgery on the TV monitor. There is no blood or guts. I can point out areas of your knee on which I'm working, making it easier for you to understand. Instead of just telling you that you had a lot of arthritis or a little, I can show you on the monitor where the arthritis is, how much you have, and how severe it is. It's better than the Discovery Channel!

---

42   Jesus Lozano, Chunbong Benjamin Ma, and W. Dilworth Cannon, "All-inside meniscus repair: A systematic review," *Clinical Orthopaedics and Related Research* 455, (February 2007): 134-141, https://doi.org/10.1097/BLO.0b013e31802ff806

After surgery, you will feel great because you still will have a lot of Novocain in your knee. You won't need crutches, but don't be fooled—the more you do on the day of surgery, the more pain you have will have the next day. So I would like you to stay on the couch, ice and elevate your knee, and only walk to the kitchen for meals, to the bathroom, and to bed. Keep bending your knee, back and forth, all day long. Remember what it's like to be in the movie theater sitting for a few hours and your knee gets stiff? Before you get up and walk, you have to bend it back and forth a few times to "lube it up." After a knee scope, all the natural lubricant is gone and replaced by saline, which isn't a good lubricant. Your natural lubrication doesn't return for several days, so it takes only five to ten minutes for your knee to stiffen up after an arthroscopy. So "lube it up" after surgery. By the next day or two, you should be feeling well.

If I do your surgery on a Friday, I expect you to be back in school or back in the office on Monday. If you are a laborer, you will return to light duty work after one week and full duty in two to three weeks.

#3 ACL Tear

Connecting the femur to the tibia, the ACL is the main stabilizing ligament of the knee and one of its most commonly injured ligaments. Immediately after the ACL is torn, you experience pain, swelling, and instability of the knee, with loss of motion and difficulty walking. Your knee gives out; you don't trust your knee. Unless you are extremely inactive and your knee doesn't give out on you with exercise or daily activity, I recommend surgical correction for ACL tears in most patients.

ACL tears never heal themselves and are rarely repairable. They shred like spaghetti. Reconstruction of the ligament is necessary, using either an autograft (your own tissue) or an allograft (tissue from a cadaver). In the literature, there is little or no difference in outcomes between the two, except maybe in varsity athletes, in whom autografts may have fewer re-tears.[43]

If I were to have an ACL reconstruction, I would choose an allograft. Since my own tissue would not be harvested, it would be less painful, and I could return to work sooner. However, if one of my children would need an ACL reconstruction, I would choose an autograft for them. Not because I would want them to have more pain than me, but because there is no risk of them acquiring any communicable diseases with an autograft. The risk of contracting HIV from an allograft is less than 1 in 1.5 million. However, when I was in medical school, we didn't even know what HIV was. So why take a risk of transferring an as-yet-unknown communicable disease to my children when we don't have to? If you are somewhere in age between me and my children and are having an ACL reconstruction, I would let you choose between an allograft and autograft.

Before surgery, a physical therapist ensures that you have full knee range of motion and that the pain and swelling have resolved. Even though that means the surgery would be two to three weeks after the initial injury, your rehab after surgery is quicker because you don't have to suffer the pain and swelling from surgery on top of the pain and swelling from the injury.

Anesthesia is general, with a nerve block to your knee. That allows for less anesthesia medication during surgery, which is always a good idea, and less need for narcotics after surgery.

Surgery is arthroscopic, through three small holes in the knee: one for the scope, one for the instrumentation, and one to harvest

---

43   Shun-Li Kan et al., "Autograft versus allograft in anterior cruciate ligament reconstruction: A meta-analysis with trial sequential analysis," *Medicine (Baltimore)* 95, no. 38 (September 2016), https://doi.org/10.1097/MD.0000000000004936

and insert the graft. You go home the same day with an ice machine that cools and compresses your knee, helping control the pain, along with a continuous passive motion (CPM) machine to restore the range of motion quickly. You are expected to go back to school or to a sedentary job two to three days afterwards, usually with crutches for one to two weeks and a brace for up to four weeks after surgery.

Our therapy program is aggressive. You begin the day after surgery with gentle range-of-motion exercises and modalities such as electrical stimulation and cold laser therapy to decrease your pain and swelling. Exercises are progressed as tolerated, getting you back to your sport as quickly and as safely as possible. However, we don't recommend contact sports until approximately six months after surgery because you may be more prone to re-tearing your ACL if you return too soon. Also, because an autograft ACL takes one year and an allograft takes 1.5 years to fully incorporate into the knee, I recommend wearing an ACL brace for sports for one and 1.5 years, respectively.[44]

Unfortunately, some patients who have had ACL tears develop arthritis in their knees later in life. Although I cannot guarantee you won't get arthritis in your knee, if I fix your ACL, I believe the arthritis won't be as bad as it would be if your knee kept on giving out, swelling, and damaging the cartilage for the next twenty years.

Once again, finding and treating the source of the ACL tear, using the methods described in this book, will speed recovery and lessen the chance of having a future injury.

---

44 Rob P.A. Janssen and Sven U. Scheffler, "Intra-articular remodeling of hamstring tendon grafts after anterior cruciate ligament reconstruction," *Knee Surgery, Sports Traumatology, Arthoscopy* 22, no. 9 (2014): 2102-2108, https://doi.org/10.1007/s00167-013-2634-5

#4 Shoulder Dislocations and Labral Tears

The management of first-time traumatic shoulder dislocations remains controversial in the orthopaedic literature. Depending on the age and activity level, there is a 30 to 75 percent chance of having a recurrent dislocation with conservative care.[45] In a study of active-duty military personnel between the ages of eighteen and twenty-six with first-time shoulder dislocations, 75 percent had a recurrent dislocation with conservative care and only 10 percent had a recurrent dislocation after surgical repair.[46] In a study of 229 patients forty years-old and younger with a twenty-five year follow-up, a study found a recurrence rate of 72 percent in patients from twelve to twenty-two years old, 56 percent in patients from twenty-three to twenty-nine years old and 27 percent in patients older than thirty.[47]

In a series of twenty-nine patients over the age of sixty with first-time dislocations, twenty-two (76 percent) had a simultaneous rotator cuff tear while nine (31 percent) had a recurrent dislocation. Only four patients (14 percent) required surgery—only one patient with a rotator cuff tear.[48] I usually like to treat my older patients with first-time shoulder dislocations with conservative care first

---

45 SM Sedeek et al., "First-time anterior shoulder dislocations: should they be arthroscopically stabilised?" *Singamore Medical Journal* 55, no. 10 (October 2014): 511-516, https://doi.org/10.11622/smedj.2014132

46 Craig R. Bottoni et a., "A Prospective, Randomized Evaluation of Arthroscopic Stabilization versus Nonoperative Treatment in Patients with Acute, Traumatic, First-Time Shoulder Dislocations," *American Journal of Sports Medicine* 30, no. 4 (July–August 2002): 576-80, https://doi.org/10.11 77/03635465020300041801

47 Lennart Hovelius et al., "Nonoperative treatment of primary anterior shoulder dislocation in patients forty years of age and younger. A prospective twenty-five-year follow-up," *Journal of Bone and Joint Surgery* 90, no. 5 (May 2008): 945-52, https://doi.org/ 10.2106/JBJS.G.00070.

48 Jose M. Rapariz et al., "Shoulder dislocation in patients older than 60 years of age," *International Journal of Shoulder Surgery* 4, no. 4 (October–December 2010): 88–92, https://doi.org/10.4103/0973-6042.79792

and see how the rotator cuff functions after the shoulder heals. But remember, every case is unique, so the rules may change accordingly.

In general, I take a more conservative approach to treating patients with first-time dislocations, except in young, high performance athletes who have a higher rate of recurrent dislocations. For a young athlete, I first will order an MRI to see if there was any structural damage to the shoulder; i.e., a large glenoid fracture or SLAP lesion. If so, he or she may require surgical correction sooner rather than later. If not, I immobilize the shoulder for one to two weeks until the pain subsides and then begin an aggressive strengthening program to strengthen the shoulder stabilizing muscles. When the strength is better than normal, the athlete may safely return to sports with a protective shoulder brace. If the athlete is unable to return to sports or cannot play at 100 percent performance, I will proceed with surgical stabilization.

For my older athletes and non-athletes, if you dislocate your shoulder in a freak accident, then consider rehabbing your shoulder and moving on with your life without surgery. I recommend a sling for the first few weeks and immediate physical therapy, including gentle, active-assisted, range-of-motion exercises, keeping your hands between your nose and your toes. Then progress to a strengthening and balance training program to decrease your chances of having another dislocation.

If you have a second dislocation, recommendation of surgery depends on the timing and mechanism of the second injury. If it was within the first six weeks of the original injury, you really didn't give the first injury enough time to heal. I consider that to be a consequence of the first dislocation and not a recurrent dislocation. If it happened in another freak accident several months or years after the first dislocation, I would recommend repeating the rehab process all over again. But if it happened after a simple, everyday task like putting on your jacket, raising your arm, or reaching into the back seat of your car, I would recommend surgery to stabilize your shoulder.

If you are loose or "double-jointed," that is, if you can do any weird tricks with your arms and hands or hyperextend your knees, elbows, wrists, and/or fingers, I strongly would recommend conservative care to strengthen your surrounding muscles to help keep your shoulder in place. Chances are that after surgically fixing your shoulder, your ligaments would just loosen up over time and probably dislocate again anyway.

Now, if you are not progressing well in rehab and have considerable shoulder pain, catching, locking, or loss of motion, or if you have a demanding physical job that requires a lot of lifting, I recommend an MRI of the shoulder looking for a labral tear and surgical correction of the shoulder sooner rather than later.

If you do have surgery, it is a same-day procedure in the hospital. The anesthesiologist gives a shot to numb the shoulder before putting you to sleep. That means less anesthesia during surgery and no pain twelve to twenty-four hours after surgery. Still, pain medication must be taken immediately after surgery to ensure adequate medication in your system before the block wears off. It's much better to stay on top of the pain rather than have to catch up with it.

An ice machine after surgery is used to decrease the pain and swelling in the shoulder, and a CPM machine helps keep the shoulder moving. The machine gently and slowly moves your shoulder as you sit in a chair, three to four times a day. At first, the motion is limited, but as you get more comfortable in the machine, the motion gradually progresses until you have full range of motion, which is expected within six weeks of surgery. Gentle physical therapy also begins immediately after surgery and progresses as tolerated. During the first six weeks, therapy focuses on isometric exercises and getting your motion back. Then it moves on to a progressive resistive exercise program over the next six weeks. You should be doing well after the first three months, but full recovery could take six months to one year after surgery. I believe in an aggressive yet well-controlled physical therapy program to ensure a rapid and safe recovery.

#5 Rotator Cuff Tear

The rotator cuff is a group of four muscles and tendons that stabilize your shoulder, allowing you to lift and rotate your arm. Rotator cuff tears can cause pain and weakness in the shoulder and difficulty lifting the arm. Many times, patients complain of shoulder pain being worse at night. While corticosteroid injections may relieve shoulder pain, they also increase the risk of subsequent rotator cuff tears and delay healing.

Generally, rotator cuff tears are seen in people over fifty years old, smokers, and overhead workers. Rotator cuff tears rarely occur in younger patients. Actually, the rotator cuff rarely "tears"; rather, it pulls away from the bone, so patients with osteoporosis and vitamin D deficiencies have more rotator cuff tears, as well as more recurrent tears after surgery.

Many people with rotator cuff tears don't even know they have a tear. In fact, there is no correlation between the size of a rotator cuff tear and the amount of pain someone experiences.[49] You can have a small rotator cuff tear and a lot of pain or a large rotator cuff tear and very little pain. Research has found the severity of pain you may experience with a rotator cuff tear is associated with your comorbidities (other things that may be wrong with you, such as diabetes, heart

---

49 Warren R. Dunn et al., "Symptoms of Pain Do Not Correlate with Rotator Cuff Tear Severity," *Journal of Bone and Joint Surgery* 96, no. 10 (May 21, 2014): 793–800, https://doi.org/10.2106/JBJS.L.01304.

disease, and back pain). I have found that patients with rotator cuff tears and one or more of the following comorbidities have the most pain: CTS, cubital tunnel syndrome, TMD, posterior rib subluxation, back pain (with or without associated obstructed breathing), and pelvic tilting (see chapters two through four).

Sleep apnea may be the reason why people with rotator cuff tears have so much more pain while sleeping. Some doctors believe waking up at nighttime with shoulder pain is a strong indicator to fix the shoulder. I recommend diagnosing and treating sleep apnea first.

So, when do I operate on patients with rotator cuff tears? I operate on them after I find and treat all comorbidities and after conservative care, including physical therapy and injections, fails to relieve their pain. I also operate on patients with rotator cuff tears who have high-demand jobs, with heavy lifting and overhead work, and on patients who cannot perform their daily routines, with or without pain or discomfort. I once operated on a spirited, healthy ninety-year-old lady with a recent rotator cuff tear who could not comb her hair. Conservative care didn't work. My colleagues thought I was nuts, but she insisted and was very grateful afterward.

Rehab after rotator cuff surgery is similar to rehab after shoulder dislocation surgery, except you may be in a sling for a longer or shorter amount of time depending on the size of the rotator cuff tear, the quality of the rotator cuff, and the quality of the bone to which it is affixed.

#6 Hip Fractures

In general, all fractures have their own personalities. Some fractures need to be fixed, while others don't. How do you know what to do? It depends. For instance, is the fracture a small, nondisplaced crack in the bone, or is it displaced and in a lot of pieces? What bone is fractured, and where on the bone is the fracture? How active is the patient? What is the quality of the bone?

However, there is little debate when it comes to hip fractures. Unless the patient is extremely ill and would die if he or she had surgery, all hip fractures should be fixed. Even if the patient never walks and is confined to a wheelchair, he or she would not be able to sit up to eat, go to the bathroom, or even roll over in bed. Because of the high risk of bed sores, pneumonia, blood clots, and unrelenting pain, it is more drastic not to operate on a patient with a hip fracture than it is to operate on him or her.

It is extremely important to quickly stabilize and take the patient to surgery as soon as possible to avoid complications of waiting too long.

Depending on the fracture and the patient, we can fix the hip with a pin, plate, or rod; replace the ball only; or replace the ball and socket of the hip. No matter how a hip fracture is fixed, the most important part of the procedure is getting the patient up and moving quickly and preventing any future fractures.

AMNRT testing and correction will improve patients' balance and outcomes. That is especially important when they are going to the bathroom in the middle of the night, in the dark, and are in danger of falling. In addition, identifying and treating sleep apnea will reduce the chance of patients getting up to go to the bathroom in the first place. Furthermore, we screen for and treat vitamin D deficiency so patients' bones will be stronger and won't break the next time they fall. Finally, we recommend they consider moving to a condo or assisted living unit where they don't have to go up and down stairs, mow the grass, or shovel the snow. The last recommendation usually falls on deaf ears, so over the years, I've learned to compromise—move the laundry room and the bedroom to the first floor.

#7 Ankle Fractures

If you fall and hurt your ankle and can't walk on it afterward, then it needs to be X-rayed. If it turns out to be broken, what do you do?

The ankle joint is made up of three bones: the fibula, the tibia, and the talus. The talus is a square bone sitting underneath and between the tibia and fibula in a sort of ring. If only one bone is broken and not displaced, the ring is stable. You usually can walk on the ankle with a fracture boot without much difficulty. The fracture should heal on its own within six weeks.

If the tibia and fibula are both broken and displaced, then the ring is unstable, and surgical correction is necessary. The joint has to line up perfectly to distribute the weight evenly, or else it could cause severe arthritis down the road. Setting the fracture and putting the ankle in a cast isn't enough; if the fracture heals in a poor position, nothing can be done about it short of rebreaking and resetting the bone, and that's a difficult operation with limited chance of success. The bottom line is that the best time to fix a displaced ankle fracture is at the time of the injury, and it should be done surgically, with plates and screws.

If there is a lot of swelling in the ankle, which often occurs, it is best to delay the surgery for a few days while icing and elevating the ankle so the swelling goes down enough to make it safe to proceed with surgery.

After surgery, I put the ankle in a fracture boot, which can be removed several times a day to work on range-of-motion exercises. Swelling and loss of motion delays recovery, so it is best to keep the leg elevated and move it as much as possible.

The amount of weight that can be placed on the repaired ankle depends on the fracture type, quality of the bone, and the strength of the hardware. Each patient with a fracture is assessed independently. Again, balance and bone strength are important in getting you moving again quickly and preventing future injuries.

#8 Wrist Fractures

The radius and the ulna are the two bones in the forearm. The distal end of the radius, the larger of the two bones at the wrist, is the most commonly fractured bone of the arm. Usually this fracture is treated with closed reduction (setting the fracture in place without surgery) and casting. However, if the fracture is severely comminuted, markedly displaced, or goes into the joint space, surgical correction is necessary.

The fracture is set into place and fixed with a plate and screws. Therapy begins early to keep the fingers moving and progresses, as the fracture heals, to increase strength.

Once again, using AMNRT testing to find and correct the problem that caused the fall in the first place is essential in preventing future falls. At the same time, diagnosing and treating osteoporosis is equally important in preventing future fractures in the event of another fall.

#9 Carpal Tunnel Surgery

Before I became familiar with AMNRT, I used to perform thirty to fifty carpal tunnel surgeries a year. In the United States, there are four to five hundred thousand carpal tunnel surgeries performed each year.[50] According to the American Board of Orthopaedic Surgery, carpal tunnel surgery is the third most common procedure performed

---

50 Craig Rodner et al., "Carpal Tunnel Syndrome," *American Academy of Orthopaedic Surgeons* 7, no. 5 (May 2009), https://www.aaos.org/OKOJ/vol7/issue5/HAN006/

by orthopaedic surgeons behind knee and shoulder arthroscopies.[51]

Although surgical outcomes are good to excellent in approximately 70 to 90 percent of patients,[52] 10 to 30 percent have persistent pain, numbness and weakness, and 8 percent of patients actually are worse after surgery.[53] Furthermore, the recurrence rate of CTS after surgery is 7 to 20 percent, and, not surprisingly, revision surgical outcomes are less successful.[54]

CTS represents a high percentage of workers' compensation (WC) claims. After surgery, compared to the normal population, WC patients took almost five weeks longer to return to work, were 16 percent less likely to return to the same level of work, and had lower functional scores. They also had nearly three times the number of complications and nearly twice the rate of persistent pain.[55]

So, avoiding carpal tunnel surgery may be a good idea. Now that I can readily find and correct the source of CTS, my patients who suffer with CTS enjoy excellent outcomes without surgery. Typically, I now do only one to two carpal tunnel surgeries a year. These are usually for patients who have had CTS for a long time where the

51   William E. Garrett et al., "American Board of the Orthopaedic Surgery Practice of the Orthopaedic Surgeon," Journal of Bone and Joint Surgery 88, no. 3 (March 2006): 660–667, https://doi.org/10.2106/00004623-200603000-00027

52   RA Brown et al., "Carpal tunnel release. A Prospective, randomized assessment of open and endoscopic methods," Journal of Bone and Joint Surgery 75, no. 9 (1993): 1265–1275, https://www.ncbi.nlm.nih.gov/pubmed/8408148

53   Jeremy D. Bland, "Treatment of carpal tunnel syndrome," Muscle & Nerve 36, no. 2 (August 2007): 167–171, https://doi.org/10.1002/mus.20802

54   Craig Rodner et al., "Carpal Tunnel Syndrome," American Academy of Orthopaedic Surgeons 7, no. 5 (May 2009), https://www.aaos.org/OKOJ/vol7/issue5/HAN006/

55   JC Dunn et al., "Outcomes Folowing Carpal Tunnel Release in Patients Receiving Workers' Compensation: A Systematic Review," HAND (New York, NY), April 2017, https://doi.org/10.1177/1558944717701240

muscle is atrophied, the sensation is gone, and the pain is severe. With surgery in these extreme cases, the pain should subside, but the weakness and numbness may persist.

I am hoping that in the future, with a large acceptance of my methods, carpal tunnel surgery will be rarely necessary.

Surgery, at times, is necessary to get you up on your feet and back into the game. Being prepared both physically and mentally for surgery is essential. In the appendix, I have included a list of thirteen ways to reduce your surgical risks and optimize your results. Follow the advice in this chapter and my tips in the appendix. If you have any questions or concerns, write them down and discuss them with your physician.

MAKING THE CORRECT DIAGNOSIS IS MOST IMPORTANT

J ake, a fifty-year-old bus driver, was turning a corner when he suddenly experienced severe shoulder pain. Even though the MRI did not show a rotator cuff tear or any other significant injury, he had three shoulder surgeries over the next eighteen months. But his pain never got better. After two years, he was placed on total disability. On the urging of a friend, he finally came to Romano Orthopaedic Center. He was soft-spoken and, I could see in his eyes, in a lot of pain. He had limited range of motion in his shoulder, with seven-out-of-ten pain.

The first thing I did was test his balance. It was off with his eyes closed. Bingo—he had CTS. He reported he had complained all the time about pain and numbness in his hand, but his orthopae-dist had ignored him. I gave him an injection for his carpal tunnel that relieved his pain by about 50 percent. Next, he had tenderness and spasticity in his lower back—again, he told me his orthopaedist refused to address his lower back. He told Jake that workers' comp only covered his shoulder, not his back or hand. So, the orthopaedist only treated his shoulder—and not successfully. When I gave Jake a shot in his lower back, he immediately began to cry. I thought I had done something wrong until he was able to compose himself and said through tears of joy, "My pain is gone!"

Making the correct diagnosis and providing expert treatment is important in surgery. But you have to go beyond that. Finding the source of the problem—understanding how you got the problem in the first place, correcting it at the source, and preventing it from recurring—is essential for a complete recovery.

What I have shown you in this book is the process I use to find the true source of an injury. Now, I don't expect you to be able to pass your orthopaedic boards after reading my book, but I do hope you have a better understanding that your injury may not be simply bad luck. It may be the result or manifestation of a separate injury or a series of injuries elsewhere. The source of your injury may be nowhere near your presenting complaint.

Balance is the key to staying healthy. If you have an injury, you will be off-balance.

You don't have to learn my techniques to diagnose your problem. Assume you have every problem listed in my book. Before you go to your orthopaedist for your back, hip, knee, shoulder, or anything similar, first try the "Romano Stretches" to relieve pain, restore your balance, improve your strength and flexibility, and prevent injuries.

"Romano Stretches"

- Kneel down with the top of your feet flat on the floor and sit back on your heels (see page 33).

- Lie on your back, bring your right knee to your left shoulder, and then across your chest. Hold for a slow count of three. Repeat with your left leg (see page 48).

- Stand up, place your right lower leg on the seat of a chair and lean back to stretch your hip flexors. Hold for a slow count of three. To get a deeper stretch, slowly bend your left knee and dip down. Repeat with your left leg on the chair (see page 64).

- Stand up and pull on your right wrist as you rotate your pelvis to the left side. Hold for a slow count of three. Repeat this stretch by pulling on your left wrist and rotating your pelvis to the right (see pages 37 and 74).

- Slowly flex your elbows to 90 degrees and then fling your elbows straight down towards the floor to quickly straighten your elbow (see page 41).

- Bring your shoulders up and keep your elbows parallel to the ground (forearms pointed forward), then fling your shoulders backwards (see page 46).

- Put both fists behind the small of your back, and then arch your back as far as you can (see page 65).

For more about the Romano Stretches, please visit
www.DrVictorRomano.com/RomanoStretches.

Don't forget: Your breathing, back, and balance are all connected. Be sure your nasal passages are fully open—not just okay. Use a nasal spray or nasal rinse, and see an ENT specialist, if necessary.

If your sleeping is interrupted by going to the bathroom during the night or because of shoulder or back pain, don't just jump to the conclusion that you drink too much water or that your pain is from moving wrong. Get checked for sleep apnea. It could save your life.

Concentrate on your nutrition and bone health. Take vitamin D, and get plenty of calcium in your diet. Don't break a bone. It's not fun.

If you do go to an orthopaedist, don't be afraid to ask him or her all the questions you need so you have a clear and thorough understanding of your diagnosis, treatment options, and treatment plan. Look for an orthopaedic surgeon who is compassionate and caring and, most importantly, who knows when to operate and when not to operate.

Stay Balanced!
Dr. Romano

APPENDIX

TOP THIRTEEN WAYS TO REDUCE YOUR SURGICAL RISKS AND OPTIMIZE YOUR RESULTS

Surgery is risky business. Fortunately, surgical complications are rare, but they are a real possibility. Many health conditions can affect the outcome of surgery. The best way to minimize your risk of complications and optimize your results is to be in the best shape possible before surgery. The following recommendations are to get you in the best shape before you proceed with any elective surgery.

1. Quit smoking.

Everyone knows that smoking leads to chronic obstructive pulmonary disease, lung cancer, heart disease, and strokes, but few people realize that smoking greatly increases the risk for complications with anesthesia and surgery.[56] Compared to nonsmokers, smokers have a higher incidence of pneumonia, blood clots, infections, pulmonary embolism (blood clot in the lung), poor wound and fracture healing, heart attacks, strokes, and death. They also have an increased risk

---

56   "Smoking and Anesthesia," American Society of Anesthesiologists, https://www.asahq.org/whensecondscount/patients%20home/ preparing%20for%20surgery/surgery%20risks/smoking%20and%20 anesthesia.

of postoperative infections, failed rotator cuff repairs, and increased loosening of total joint replacements.

Quitting smoking six to eight weeks before an elective surgery is the single most important thing you can do to decrease your risk of developing postoperative complications and improve your chances for a successful surgical outcome. Even quitting twenty-four hours before surgery is better than smoking just before surgery. Do not resume smoking for several weeks afterwards. Better yet, stop smoking altogether.

Nicotine replacement therapy, such as gums, lozenges, and patches, can double your chances of quitting for good, but you need more. Develop a strategy to quit smoking and pick a start date. Go to smokefree.gov for a great start.

2. Lose weight and improve nutrition.

Compared to normal-weight patients, obese patients (BMI> 30)[*] generally have more problems with surgery. Because of their body habitus (type), surgery is more technically challenging in obese patients, increasing their time spent in surgery. Anesthesia is also more difficult to administer. Locating veins, ensuring sufficient oxygen and airflow, and properly positioning the needle when delivering spinal and epidural nerve blocks or other types of regional anesthesia can be a problem. Morbidly obese patients (BMI > 40) have an extremely high risk of complications, so much so that total joint replacements are not advisable.[57] These surgical complications include the following:

---

[*] Body mass index (BMI) is the measurement of body fat based on height and weight. BMI = Weight (lb) / [Height (in)]² x 703

57 Ryan Martin, Jason Jennings, and Douglas Dennis, "Morbid Obesity and Total Knee Arthroplasty: A Growing Problem," *Journal of the American Academy of Orthopaedic Surgeons* 25, no. 3 (March 2017): 188–194, https://doi.org/10.5435/JAAOS-D-15-00684.

- Infection
- Poor wound healing
- Blood clots
- Pulmonary embolism
- Failed surgeries

Whether you are overweight or not, you can have poor nutritional health, which leads to wound infections and delayed healing. We routinely assess your nutrition. Improving your nutritional status and losing weight will decrease your complication risk and increase the likelihood of having a successful surgical outcome. Before undergoing an elective orthopaedic procedure, consider making the following key lifestyle changes:

- **Reduce fat and calorie intake**. Eat a well-balanced, nutritious diet that includes plenty of fresh fruits and vegetables, whole grains, lean meats, and low-fat dairy. Eliminate unnecessary carbohydrates. Drink plenty of water, and avoid high-calorie, sugary drinks. A good rule of thumb is, no matter how big your dinner plate is, fill one-quarter of it with protein—chicken, pork, grass-fed beef, or fish. Fill the remaining three-quarters with vegetables— the more color, the better.

- **Increase daily physical activity and exercise**. The better shape you are in before surgery, the quicker your recovery. Constant hip or knee pain may make you less active than you were before. If you have arthritis, low-impact activities— such as swimming, biking, or using an elliptical machine— will limit the stress on your joints, so you can exercise comfortably to help you lose weight more effectively. In addition, there is a chance losing weight may decrease your pain enough that you no longer need a joint replacement, or at least allow you to put it off for years.

3. Control your diabetes.

People with poorly controlled diabetes are at a higher risk of postoperative complications, including infection, wound complications, silent heart attacks (you don't feel them), and kidney failure. HbA1c is a blood marker that correlates with how well a patient's sugars have been controlled over the past month. Patients with HbA1c over seven have had poorly controlled diabetes over that last month and thus are at a higher risk of complications.

Furthermore, if you are on insulin, surgery will cause increased stress to your body and raise your blood sugar, so your insulin dose may need to be adjusted. If you have diabetes and your HbA1c is over seven, talk to your primary care provider about the best way to control your blood sugar—and to a nutritionist to optimize your diet—before proceeding with surgery.

4. Practice good dental hygiene.

Every time you get your teeth cleaned, there may be a little or a lot of bleeding from your gums, depending on your oral health. Bacteria from your mouth can then get into your bloodstream and settle on total joint prostheses, causing an infection. If you are having a surgery requiring any sort of implant, visit your dentist to clean your teeth and to take care of any necessary dental work before surgery. If you have a joint replacement and have poorly controlled diabetes or are immunocompromised, the American Academy of Orthopaedic Surgeons and the American Dental Association recommend that you take antibiotics before each teeth cleaning.[58]

---

58 Ayesha Abdeen et al., "Appropriate Use Criteria For the Management of Patients with Orthopaedic Implants Undergoing Dental Procedures,"

5. See your cardiologist.

If you have a history of coronary artery disease, congestive heart failure, or atrial fibrillation (abnormal heart rhythm), visit your cardiologist for clearance before surgery. These conditions can place you at far greater risk of life-threatening complications during and for months after surgery.

6. Screen for sleep apnea.

It's estimated that up to 25 percent of people may have sleep apnea, although 80 to 90 percent go undiagnosed.[59] Patients with sleep apnea who have total joint replacements are 44 percent more likely to have complications compared to patients without sleep apnea. If you normally aren't breathing well during sleep, anesthesia and pain medication both can further depress your breathing, leading to heart attacks, strokes, and even death.

If anyone has noticed that you snore loudly and hold your breath while sleeping, or if you ever have fallen asleep at a long stoplight, you should be tested for sleep apnea right away with a take-home or in-lab sleep study. You also should be tested for sleep apnea if you have a high score on the Epworth Sleepiness Scale (available online), which rates your likelihood of falling asleep while watching TV, reading a book, talking to a friend, being a passenger in a car, and at other times.

Before surgery, patients with sleep apnea should see a sleep specialist to receive a CPAP machine or a dentist specializing in sleep apnea to be fitted with an oral appliance to control sleep apnea.

American Academy of Orthopaedic Surgeons and American Dental Association, 2016, https://www.aaos.org/downloadasset.aspx?id=4294971319.

59 Kingman P. Strohl, "Patient education: Sleep apnea in adults (Beyond the Basics)," UpToDate, last updated November 6, 2017, https://www.uptodate.com/contents/sleep-apnea-in-adults-beyond-the-basics.

7. Improve your bone health.

Before total joint replacement, we recommend a bone density exam along with bone health lab tests that measure calcium and vitamin D levels to determine the quality of your bones. Patients with untreated osteoporosis have a higher risk of loosening of the prosthesis and greater revision rate.[60] Maximizing your bone health will improve your results.

8. Limit your alcohol intake.

More than two drinks per day can lead to alcohol abuse, with associated elevated liver function tests, increased perioperative bleeding and blood transfusions, longer hospital stays, higher complication rate, and a fifteen times higher risk of postoperative infection and death.

It pays to be honest about your drinking before surgery. Careful control of pain medication, more frequent postoperative visits, and/ or inpatient postoperative rehab will help you get through the surgery without alcohol.

9. Seek help for anxiety and depression.

Understandably, patients who have considerable pain and difficulties with daily activities may also have some degree of anxiety and depression. Because they often are not motivated to do the necessary rehabilitation, patients with anxiety and depression can have an increased dependence on opioid pain medication after surgery and a slower and incomplete recovery.[61] To optimize your surgical results, you need to be both physically and mentally prepared. If you have symptoms of anxiety and/or depression, seek professional help before surgery.

---

60   Jin Kyu Lee and Choong-Hyeok Choi, "Total Knee Arthoplasty in Rheumatoid Arthritis," *Knee Surgery & Related Research* 24, no. 1 (March 2012): 1-6, https://doi.org/10.5792/ksrr.2012.24.1.1

61   Martin Cheadle et al., "Treating Pain in Addicted Patients: Recommendations from an Expert Panel," *Population Health Management* 17, no. 2 (April 2014): 79-89, https://doi.org/10.1089/pop.2013.0041

10. Stop arthritis and pain medication.

If you are on arthritis medication before surgery, it is important you stop the medication at least one week before the procedure. Anti-inflammatory medication may cause excessive bleeding that can be harmful after surgery. Stopping the medication with enough time before surgery lessens these side effects.

Patients who are on medications for rheumatoid arthritis need to stop them several weeks or more before surgery. These medications inhibit the body's natural inflammatory response, putting the patient at an increased risk of postoperative infections and delayed healing.

Regular use of narcotic medication to control your orthopaedic pain before surgery can make it harder to control pain after surgery. Furthermore, chronic use of narcotic medication can lead to post-operative complications.[62] Withdrawal from narcotics can lead to seizures and confusion. Talk with your doctor about how to decrease or stop your opioid medication before surgery. Consulting a pain specialist may be necessary to help you control your opioid use.

11. Clean your skin and nose.

Clean and healthy skin is essential for wound healing. Do not shave the skin over the planned surgical site for two weeks prior to surgery. For five days before and on the morning of surgery, shower daily with over-the counter chlorhexidine antibiotic soap and leave a thin film on the skin. This will decrease the bacteria count of the skin and lessen your risk of a surgical site infection (SSI). You also should use this soap to wash your hands and to protect your incision when you come home after surgery.

---

62 Ingrid Hein, "Presurgical Opioids Heighten Addiction Risk, Complications," Medscape, last modified March 4, 2016, https://www.medscape.com/viewarticle/859871

Methicillin-resistant Staphylococcus aureus (MRSA) infections are no longer limited to the hospital and are an ever-growing problem in the community. One out of five patients have the Staphylococcus bacteria growing in their nasal passage without any symptoms.[63] I recommend all patients undergoing total joint replacements swab their nose twice a day with an antibiotic ointment to remove colonization of MRSA and decrease their SSI risk.

12. Screen for anemia.

Patients who are anemic (have a low red blood cell count) before surgery are at a higher risk of having more complications, including perioperative strokes and heart attacks. They also are at an increased risk of receiving blood transfusions. With each blood transfusion, there is an increased risk of infection. So it is important to check the blood cell count before surgery. If the blood level is low, we refer the patient back to their primary care physician to determine the cause; it may be that they are losing blood through an ulcer in the stomach or for some other reason. If the cause is simply low iron intake, we give iron and vitamin C pills to increase the red blood cell level so the surgery can proceed safely. We may also give an injection of a synthetic hormone to increase the blood level faster.

13. Get your body and home in shape for surgery.

To get the best results from surgery, it is important to be in the best shape ahead of time. Total joint replacement patients are started on a pre-operative, supervised, home exercise program to increase their core

---

63   ME Mulcahy et al., "Nasal Colonisation by Staphylococcus aureus Depends upon Clumping Factor B Binding to the Squamous Epithelial Cell Envelope Protein Loricrin," *PLOS Pathogens* 8, no. 12 (December 2012): e1003092, https://doi.org/10.1371/journal.ppat.1003092

strength, flexibility, and balance. We also send a specialist to their home environment to ensure it is safe for them to return soon after surgery or to see if in-house therapy is a better option. The specialist may also recommend safety tips like installing grab bars in the bathroom and removing throw rugs that may be a tripping hazard.

OUR PILLARS OF SERVICE

At Romano Orthopaedic Center, our guiding philosophies are quite simple: Do what's right for the patient; do our best to avoid surgery if possible; and when surgery is necessary, ensure that the patient has the right preparation for surgery and the right care post-surgery. Romano Orthopaedic Center takes a holistic approach to medicine and patient care. For over twenty-five years, we have taken care of general orthopaedic ailments for the Greater Chicago area, from kids to the elderly. For more information on the practice, visit www.RomanoMD.com.

Nine pillars of services offered:

- Sports medicine
- Total joint replacements
- Fracture care
- Bone and joint health
- Sleep apnea and breathing problems
- Physical therapy
- Balance, stability, and flexibility
- Injury prevention
- Nutrition